WRESTLING WITH GHOSTS

A Personal And

Scientific Account Of

Sleep Paralysis

WRESTLING WITH
GHOSTS

A Personal And
Scientific Account Of
Sleep Paralysis

JORGE CONESA SEVILLA, PH.D.

To order additional copies of this book, contact:
Xlibris Corporation
1-888-795-4274
www.Xlibris.com
Orders@Xlibris.com
23899

CONTENTS

*I dedicate this work to my wife Cindy, an ally and
source of support throughout many sleep paralysis events
and the writing of this book. I also dedicate this work to my
children Jordi, Kaliana, Patrick and Jasson. I am grateful
to our daughter Kaliana, a sleep paralysis sufferer herself,
for her help in coding some of the narratives and case reports
and for contributing her art work for the cover. I thank all
the subjects who participated in the experiments or
contributed narratives or questionnaires. Finally,
I am indebted to Ms. Lucy Gillis
for her contribution and support.*

PREFACE

This year (2004) the sleep research community celebrates 50 years since the discovery of Rapid Eye Movement Sleep (REM) by a then graduate student, E. Aserinsky (This work was published in 1955; Aserinsky, and Kleitman, 1955). Joining in this celebration and spirit of discovery this book is the first of its kind in the study of a mysterious phenomenon of REM sleep, *sleep paralysis* (SP), and also the longest case study of dream content and frequencies in the dream literature to date, certainly, when it comes to *sleep paralysis* itself. In addition to this case study, the work shares narratives and questionnaire data from independent samples. Also, this is a recent attempt to create a link between *sleep paralysis* and *lucid dreaming*. The work also prescribes practical ways of managing the fear associated with the so-called "Old Hag" experience.

I am a neurocognitive and biosemiotic researcher who has experienced sleep paralysis since 1969 and continue to experience sleep paralysis routinely. I have published my research on sleep paralysis since 1995 and recently reported the findings of a ten-year longitudinal study about this sleep syndrome, the longest study tracking sleep paralysis to date (Conesa, 1995, 1997, 200, 2002, and 2003). Given this dual background, in this book, I approach this fascinating sleep experience and resulting lucid dreams from both personal-developmental and scientific perspectives. Prior to entering graduate school and commencing this line of research, I, like many other sufferers of sleep paralysis, did not know the name or cause of these uncanny and surreal dreamscapes I experienced.

In this short book, I have attempted to summarize the scientific work about this mysterious sleep disorder, for example, looking at the commonality between the sleep paralysis and lucid dreaming experience on one hand and the so-called extraterrestrial alien abduction phenomenon on the other. While trying to explain the link between these seemingly diverse experiences, I found it necessary to revisit Freudian and Jungian dream descriptions and hypotheses, the philosophy of aesthetics and the juxtaposition of the former explanations with respect to shamanic practices and interpretations of dreaming.

Wrestling With Ghosts summarizes and updates a growing literature that includes traditional cultural accounts, scientific research, and subjective reports about the uncanny sleep disorder referred to as *sleep paralysis* (SP). The book serves, I think, as an important tool to normalize the *sleep paralysis* experience by attempting to remove its often-publicized mystical and supernatural aura. Specifically, the book is a serious contribution to the psychological and social scientific literature as an example of behavioral/social methodology in clarifying psychological phenomena that can be misinterpreted individually or by culture as "paranormal." However, the book does not refute the very real phenomenology of the experience and is intended as a practical guide for recognizing and managing the disorder in creative and self-enhancing ways. That is, the book provides sleep paralysis sufferers with practical suggestions for coping with their disorder in positive ways that induce the creative aspect of lucid dreaming by introducing the method of Sleep Paralysis Signaling (*SPS*).

In aggregate, this work reiterates the aesthetic and creative power of *uncanny dreaming* regardless of its scientific origin. This *aesthetic* dimension of sleep paralysis and lucid dreaming, perhaps the most important of all, is a juxtaposition of mythical, shamanic, creative, personal and scientific multidisciplinary approaches to studying and describing dream phenomenology.

This work provides a retrospective look at the history of this uncanny disorder in human evolution, its recent western medical history and its most recent empirical and/or phenomenological descriptions as so-called alien abduction cases, including a presentation of Jungian and Freudian mythical perspectives. The empirical data, although cumbersome at times, is a necessary part of the story I want to share with all readers, but it is presented in balance with traditional cross-cultural and folklore accounts of the disorder as well as in the context of numerous recent cases researched in conjunction with the long-term study. Included in this story, and in agreement with Persinger (1987), is a proposal about *psycho-geographical* and *psycho-geomagnetic* distributions of "ghost" stories, dream attacks, and other SP related phenomena. I have argued in print (Conesa, 2000 and 2003) that these geographical zones correlate with geodynamic areas such as the Pacific "Ring of Fire" region where an increased number of cultural names for SP and its frequencies are reported (my "ring of fire" hypothesis).

This book is written and intended for a general educated audience; anyone interested in dream phenomenology and behavior; the medical professional; folklorists; psychologists interested in dream phenomenology and behavior; sleep researchers; and the clinical psychologist. It would be a great honor if the book succeeds in continuing and expanding the scholarly work of Dr. David Hufford, who published the now classic account of sleep paralysis as Newfoundland's "Old Hag" phenomenon.

I would like to acknowledge the contributions and support of many people who directly or indirectly have made these pages possible: Ms. Lucy Gillis who contributed her lucid dreaming experiences and commentary; all my students and subjects around the world who volunteered information about their sleep paralysis/lucid dreaming condition; and the attention and generosity of Drs. Hufford, Brugger, Blackmore,

Domhoff and Takeuchi. I am thankful to Dr. Stephen LaBerge for clarifying important points about the physiology of lucid dreaming. I hope he is tolerant of my own interpretations of lucid dreaming with respect to the larger body of data presented here. I am also indebted to Dr. Coles from the Geological Survey of Canada for providing, for ten years, the *aa* indices upon which some of the data analysis depends and for invaluable help in interpreting geophysical data. Special thanks are in order to two informants about cross-cultural aspects of sleep paralysis elsewhere in the world. Specifically, I am grateful to Mr. Asmara-Winang for his contribution of *Tindihan* in Indonesia and to Mr. Rick Carroll for his contribution of the *Huaka'i po* (Night Marchers) in Hawaii. Sadly, I have misplaced other correspondence and emails related to the prevalence of sleep paralysis among the Inuit in Alaska, including reports of coping strategies and folklore. I nevertheless want to acknowledge these contributors as well and thank them for their time and correspondence.

Finally, I wish to extend my warm and heartfelt gratitude to Dr. Marcelo Murillo from Argentina for his continued correspondence and support throughout the last four years. Specifically, I am indebted to him for his ideas and interest about a possible connection between sleep paralysis episodes and early morning heart failure. This ongoing connection will no doubt be the source of future multidisciplinary research that I already look forward to.

INTRODUCTION

"There is widespread in Newfoundland a form of sleep paralysis known as the "Old Hag," or "ag rog," (Ness 1978) and in its grip one is "hagged," or "hag-ridden" (Hufford, 1976). One so afflicted finds himself unable to move but is conscious and able to hear . . . Being "hagged" is sometimes accompanied by hallucinations, such as a cat sitting upon the chest or a woman dressed in white holding one down. It is felt that it is most likely to occur to a person sleeping on his or her back. The term "Old Hag" refers both to the terrifying experience and to the entity that attacks the victim during the experience (Hufford, 1982)."

Melvin Firestone, *The "Old Hag:"*
Sleep Paralysis in Newfoundland, 1985

At this moment, I am writing at 7:45 PM and I know that I have, at most, one more hour of *wakeful lucidity* before I start falling asleep. Going to bed this early may strike some readers as a premature bedtime especially for an active and healthy male in his forties. More disturbing is the fact that when sleep comes, I, like a small percentage of individuals who experience chronic *Isolated Sleep Paralysis* (ISP or SP), expect my dream life to be terrifying, peculiar or bizarre.

Those of us who experience what David Hufford called "the terror that comes in the night," usually when falling asleep and especially if we are unusually tired, will regain and/or maintain conscious awareness and witness some of the very physiology of sleep from a personal and sometimes skewed perspective. Retaining self-awareness during a time when most dreamers are unconscious opens the door to a dreamscape of strange bodily sensations (See Appendix II) sounds, apparitions, goblins, extra-terrestrial abductors, and always the experience of paralysis, pressure or suffocation.

Additionally, imagine for a moment being a child or an adolescent experiencing these mostly nocturnal events[1] for days, weeks, or years and not being able to share these bizarre encounters for fear that people may think you mad! Throughout this book, we will explore this sleep disorder, Sleep Paralysis or Isolated Sleep Paralysis, what David Hufford and Robert Ness termed *The Old Hag*[2]. As in Hufford's seminal work, I will normalize the Old Hag experience, attempting to remove some of its supernatural aura by sharing the latest scientific and cross-cultural information about the phenomenon. However, departing from both authors, I will also present a more benign and creative aspect of the phenomenon. That is, the intensity of these experiences, their subjective reality, can also be very positive; thus the Old Hag can be turned into a beautiful princess or any other happier mentation by means of exercises that will be described in Chapter Five.

Examining in this short book the medical, mythical, cross-cultural, and practical complexities as well as the creative possibilities of this disorder is no small task. But I will begin with a summary of relevant research that looks at the psychology of this disorder in Chapters One and Two. Also, throughout the book, I will share personal accounts and the sleep paralysis experiences of our subjects and co-researchers and use these to introduce a classification of the behaviors and experiences that accompany sleep paralysis for the average sufferer[3]. Furthermore, since sleep paralysis is often associated with **Lucid Dreaming** (LD) states, I will devote a chapter (Chapter 3) to exploring this important connection but it will be a connection that I will speak of frequently throughout this book. Finally, I will share a list of recommendations of measures that can be harnessed and practiced in order to minimize the negative experiences associated with SP or to minimize the probability or their occurrence by practicing new sleep habits and rituals (In Chapters 4 and 5). And, yes, some of these rituals may include going to bed earlier than most folks.

To summarize, this book differs from other recent SP literature in at least six fundamental ways. *First*, it presents the SP phenomenon from a unique, personal, and subjective point of view as well as from an empirical and objective orientation since the roles of chronic sufferer; phenomenological experiencer; and neurocognitive researcher are folded into one person. I was (am) fully aware before I began my SP research that a perceived "conflict of interest" may make some scientists be extra cautious with the data I present. Such a reader is referred to other experimental efforts conducted by the author and asks them that they trust that the quality of this basic research training in the areas of biosemiotics, psychophysics, psychobiology and neurocognition is also applied to the study of SP. However, as an insider, I bring an unambiguous and clear impression of the power of the uncanny to seduce and to be misinterpreted and hope that my scientific training counterbalances these powerfully felt tendencies. In addition to my own experiences, I will present case studies throughout the book when appropriate, but in particular, I am pleased to highlight the LD experiences of Ms. Lucy Gillis. Her words stand on their own merit and are a wonderful example of the intricacies of dreaming as a rich and powerful phenomenology. *Second*, this book elaborates on and shares additional information on the only longitudinal SP case study, ten years, published to date. *Third*, the technique of Sleep Paralysis Signaling (*SPS*) is introduced as a natural means for cuing, inducing and controlling lucid dreaming states. *Fourth*, the incidence of SP is evaluated while introducing the purported role of global geomagnetic influences. The geomagnetic influences are falsified by a grand testable hypothesis, the "ring of fire," that there exists around the globe geophysically unstable regions (such as the Pacific, ring of fire volcanic zone) that give rise to an increase reporting of SP phenomena. These areas are what I have termed psycho-geographical or psycho-geophysical unstable zones. *Fifth*, few SP studies and reports elaborate further the often-reported role of SP in lucid dreaming. That is, many SP sufferers are also lucid dreamers in almost equal frequency. Or, individuals who lucid dream, also report having experienced SPs. And finally, *sixth*, starting in chapter two and until the end of this presentation I will go back to the ancient and classical roots, study and practice, of LD and sleep paralysis within the context of what it is referred to as "shamanism" and to the legacy of a selected number of ideas that Sigmund Freud and Carl G. Jung proposed that are still worth thinking about. We owe a great deal to both influences and stories. *This examination of shamanism-as-art, or even of shamanism-as-poetry, is proposed as a sort of compromise (between the austere-scientific and the extreme-unfounded new age proposals) and evidence that human dreamers long ago, and into the present, have developed creative and meaningful ways of coping with and extending the possibilities of self-aware dreaming states.*

But first, I will devote a few paragraphs defining some terms that researchers employ when talking about Isolated Sleep Paralysis (henceforth ISP) or terms that I tend to use interchangeably in order to prevent confusion.

Old Terms New Terms

Sleep Paralysis, henceforth abbreviated as SP[4], is the general term used to describe *being self-aware during the rapid-eye movement (REM) stage of sleep—specifically being self-aware of the loss of body muscle tone accompanying REM sleep—when we usually experience vivid dreams.* Physiologically speaking, when we dream in the REM stage of normal, uneventful sleep, our bodies are paralyzed (different than being merely lethargic) so that we cannot act out the content of our dreams. This paralysis occurs for the average normal dreamer three to four times every night for the duration of the REM stage[5]. If we live to our present-day average life expectancy of 73-75 years, roughly ten of those years would have been spent in this state of sleep paralysis. From the onset, and important to this attempt at a psychological normalization of the phenomenon, it is worth considering the fact that if we were not paralyzed during REM states and the bizarre and rich dreams that accompany this stage, we could hurt ourselves or our sleeping partners; we might even find ourselves in a situation much like that of Mr. Stephen Clay Jones, Sr., who accidentally killed his wife during a REM sleep episode. Mr. Jones suffered from a REM Sleep Disorder that disinhibited natural SP[6]. In short SP (or ISP) is self-awareness during (and of) the REM stage. This self-awareness may extend to the experience of some of the psychobiological, psychological, and physiological events occurring during these periods. All of the above circumstances have been given cultural interpretation resulting in our folklore of "The Old Hag" in Newfoundland; Pesadilla in Spanish speaking countries, Huaka'i po (Night Marchers) in Hawaii; Doppelganger in Germany; Kanashibari in Japan; Tindihan in Indonesia; ghosts in numerous cultures; and even perhaps some of the alien abduction phenomena.

Adding to a possible confusion when reading the scientific literature, the description of sleep paralysis and the use of this general term is included in a set of symptoms in other populations, such as a segment of individuals who also experience narcolepsy. Thanks to the initial observations and research of Drs. Wilson and Hishikawa looking at SP and its appearance in some narcoleptics, a great deal about the incidence of SP in the normal population was ascertained.

According to the Diagnostic and Statistical Manual of Mental Disorders, IV (TR), up to 50% of the narcoleptic population report SPs. This later clarification was aided (and continues— read about Dr. Takeuchi's latest work in Chapter 1) by the work of Drs. Hufford, Fukuda and Takeuchi. *However, the term Isolated Sleep Paralysis (ISP) is very specific to describing the same experiences in otherwise normal populations without other symptoms, even when the SP experience is a once-in-a-life time event.* For the most part, I will use the terms SP and ISP interchangeably, to mean the occurrence of these experiences in the normal population, unless I specifically refer to the scientific literature that distinguishes between the two terms.

Because I and others also use SP as a signal and launching pad, so to speak, for more creative dream experiences (Please refer to the Sleep Paralysis Signaling, *SPS*, described in Chapter 5), I have fallen into the habit of calling SP *Bound Lucidity*, a more neutral term than "The Old Hag" and less clinical than the historical connotation of SP or even ISP. Even though my preference for "Bound Lucidity" may not endure beyond its use in my own research, this phrase nevertheless reminds me that, *"The Old Hag" is only one possible experiential manifestation of ISP,* and it is very likely that future psychological and folklore studies will implicate the SP experience with more positive and mind-manifesting experiences, including so-called mystical states (out-of-the-body-experiences, bliss, and insight). I am mindful of the fact that without a disciplined management of the SP condition the negative experiences are reported in greater numbers (historically, *folklorically*, and personally), since they are most disturbing, than the positive experiences. *It makes sense since sleep is a nightly journey at the end of another one: it occurs at the end of waking experiences, some of which may be emotionally charged. Assuming that we are psychologically more vulnerable at the end of the day, consequently the dice are cast toward altering dream content toward the negative.* Unless the dreamer can affect the hours before sleep in such a way that he/she is psychologically calm and relaxed and in control of the panic associated with finding himself/herself in a state of paralysis (see Chapter 4), then the negative experiences will be more likely to occur than the positive ones. Finally, when used throughout this book, the phrase **Bound Lucidity** will be our code and reminder that SP/ISP can be used for the specific purpose of attaining Lucid Dreaming or to mitigate and control the SP state itself.

A Systematic Study of SP

Because of the very intense subjective reality of the events occurring during **Bound Lucidity**, even if a small percentage of the human population experiences chronic SP, then their stories of goblins, space visitors, astral projections, ghosts, thunderous noises as well as ethereal music, are likely to have left important historical and cultural marks. The very presence of these dreaming events within an interpretative folklore tradition serves as corroboration of reality to new generations of naïve SP sufferers. Unfortunately, the easier and often-supernatural interpretation that helps the SP sufferer to validate this phenomenon at a local, cultural level, only adds to the difficulty that these experiences may become scientifically explainable to the sufferer, some time during their lifetime. *The major obstacle to a scientific understanding of SP has to do with the relatively little medical or psychological research devoted to the disorder, and by logical extension, the lack of information that exists even within the medical establishment on how to help the SP sufferer. But a vast body of research does exists on sleep and dreaming in general, and it seems that the layperson does not understand it, or this body of knowledge has not been communicated effectively in popular books or articles. That is, this general body of information would be enough, if adequately disseminated and accessed, to elucidate some important aspects of* *the SP experience.* Perhaps as a consequence of this information vacuum and lack of generalized therapeutical interventions I have received, for example, many emails related to our scientific perspective of SP presented in our web page whose writers cannot or will not accept sleep a as a series of dynamic stages and states where REM reality and awaken reality can be fused at times. To be fair, a greater number of comments, narratives and emails are expressions of relief at having found first a label for their set of symptoms and then a scientific path zeroing in on a physiological explanation. The new research horizons of using the Internet as a dissemination tool to reach millions of readers can also be a powerful and positive force in taking the mystery out of SP phenomenology. When valid online questionnaires are employed that facilitate understanding of the SP experience, subjects have a way of normalizing their symptoms in the context of the scientific literature. I am rewarded by the fact that these individuals are extremely thankful for finding some of the answers they seek[7].

From these letters and our research and conclusions thereof, a set of four maxims can be distilled that might explain why individuals cannot accept at times the intense events of SP as part of a medically/scientifically describable sleep phenomena. At least one of these maxims also includes the philosophical and psychological insight about consciousness being a private and subjective experience.

Sleep is dynamic. The cycles and stages of sleep taking the sleeper from conscious to unconscious states can vary from person to person, from night to night, or from hour to hour in a person's individual experience, depending on environmental circumstances, or changes in lifestyle or habits. Not only is sleep dynamic but obviously consciousness itself is also dynamic, thus as consciousness and/or self-awareness changes during sleep a variety of phenomenological states are possible. *More specifically, experientially speaking, an SP* *experiencer can move from being awake, to alternate reality (dream reality with self-awareness), to sleepiness and confusion, to total unconsciousness very quickly[8]. This experiential flux opens the door, understandably, for the misinterpretation and/or admixing of the objectively real as well as dreamt images, sensations, story lines, and emotions.* This experiential vulnerability during SP should not come as a surprise since even when the average person is awake, a bit tired, overloaded with information, and expecting a specific experiential outcome, reality and memories can be manufactured so that a seemingly real, but not necessarily accurate reality is arrived at. We sit by the phone waiting the phone call from a lover and, believing that we just heard the phone ringing, pick up the receiver only to find out that it never did. Similarly, we talk about someone framing a question in a particular way so as to "lead" the witness. Finally, humans are generally speaking, prejudiced, or at least think stereotypically, and thus see the world in a subjective light regardless of information to the contrary. *In short, during sleep, and in particular during an SP episode, both external and internal realities may be rapidly stitched together into a unique experience that crosses the threshold into the uncanny and the bizarre, with all the intensity of the "real".* Finally, the dynamics of sleep for the SP experiencer often includes other salient experiences such as **Lucid Dreaming**. This leaves us with a rich experiential situation where this population of dreamers also has access to, witnessing and reporting, the quick and abrupt changes of consciousness that characterize sleep cycles and stages, as well as accessibility to many dream phenomena usually written about as stand alone experiences. The data that will be presented and the narratives shared in these pages suggest that SP experiencers are exposed to a plethora of phenomenology of dreaming that can be overwhelming for the experiencer and difficult to tease out as a researcher. But I think that once examined, the SP experience has the potential to confirm many observations that have been gathered electrophysiologically, in the more aseptic environment of the sleep laboratory, and to continue adding to the literature of dream content and quality.

Consciousness is private and subjective. The philosopher John Searle considers the subjective aspect of consciousness to be one of its salient attributes. In connection to the earlier observation of sleep as a dynamic state, the intensity of the SP experiences are always felt as REAL. And they are REAL, in a subjective sense. *That means that the SP episodes and related experiences are memorable and significant events, as important and palpable as any other event (maybe even more!) occurring in one's subjective, intimate life.* To the extent that ghosts appear, aliens come visiting, one's body floats away into other dreamscapes, AND the SP experiencer is subjectively aware of these occurrences taking place, then these will be treated as "real." Thus there will be a serious and tenacious attempt at explaining their cause and predict their future appearance. Subjective reality overrides incredulity and self-doubt in the end. Because the prominent feature of SP is being self-aware of the REM accompanying paralysis itself, which it is truly happening for all dreamers, the rest of the experience is also accepted without qualifications. Usually, the dreamer is left to interpret these occurrences on his/her own or, if lucky, within a cultural context that can "explain" these events. SP is no doubt an intimate experience. Often times, only a spouse or a significant other can assist a dreamer who experiences SP regularly. *The SP sufferer and his/her regular sleeping partner develop their own unique ways to awaken by touch, primarily, and even by learning how to distinguish that a certain moan or twitch means that their loved one is in frozen panic. But even a spouse may be doubtful and suspicious of these reports.* As an analogy, I am reminded that it is very hard to convey how painful a migraine headache can be to people who have never experienced them. It is also difficult to convey the exquisite details of and potential for controlling a lucid dream to people who rarely remember their own dreams, or when they do, only report fleeting or vague black and white impressions. At worst, if no intimate circle exists, the SP sufferer may endure these experiences alone for years before telling anyone, usually for fear that others will think him/her mad! These powerful experiences kept secret for so long have the potential of charting unusual life paths or even altering behavior significantly from day to day toward the path of dysfunction.

The cultural context "colors" the SP experience. The psychological and the cultural go hand in hand, and in the case of SP, there is convincing evidence from writers like Hufford, Hishikawa and Firestone that diverse folklore around the world, past and present, is a cultural validation of and attempt to explain universal and precise set of SP symptoms (Please refer to Appendix I.). In Hawaii SP is explained as "night marchers," the souls of ancient warriors walking in the vicinity of the sufferer. In Indonesia, Central America, Alaska, and Fiji, SP and related dreams are perceived as ghost visitations. Additionally, and in a more contemporary setting, others and myself believe that much of the so-called alien abduction phenomena, particularly when the so-called abductees report these experiences at nighttime and relate the paralysis itself, is a new twist and cultural explanation of SP. Many of these folkloric interpretations attempt to address the many components, contextual and bodily (sleeping quarters, body and head position, setting, family, local history, personality), that are part of the canonical SP experience and serve to aid the dreamer in managing or coping with his/her condition. Only when the sleep/dream researcher sets out to classify, systematize, and compare these local experiential features does a universal and psychobiological pattern emerge. At the end of this book and presentation I hope it is clear to the reader that I am in no way trying to minimize the contribution of folkloric explanations to the scientific study of SP. As Hufford observed, it is often through folklore that we can begin to explore scientifically the underpinnings of a medical, astronomical, or maritime phenomenon[9]. Thus I will employ folkloric accounts of SP as necessary data that need to be sorted out and that could potentially shed light on the phenomenon at hand in conjunction with the scientific method and study of SP. As a prelude to this juxtaposition and cooperation of folkloric and scientific data, less-written about cultural interpretations of SP, Indonesia's Tindihan or Hawaii's Night Marchers, *Huaka'i-po*, include a description of specific locations (and/or positions) where the dreamer should be in order to avoid the experiences. For example, to avoid an encounter with Huaka'i-po the dreamer should avoid falling asleep in the ancient trails that the warriors still use. In order not to be taken away, as legend prescribes, one who encounters Huaka'i-po must lay still, face down, not look at the warriors, and wait until they leave. The scientific connection I refer to is my earlier work in trying to assess a relationship between SP episodes and abrupt changes in the local geomagnetic flux[10]. Geomagnetic effects, known to have actual effects on brain structures and function, include local magnetic anomalies as well that could affect some individuals and specifically, an SP-prone dreamer. I presented what I alluded to earlier as the "ring of fire" hypothesis[11]— that countries and folklore that flourish in geomagnetically unstable regions of the world such as the vast pan Pacific Ring of Fire zone, may have a richer vocabulary and management specific to the SP experience given the fact that their populations experience these geological upheavals more frequently. In addition to these two Pacific Rim cultures of Hawaii and Indonesia, other pan Pacific locations/cultures have reported the SP experience in detail. These include the Inuit in Alaska, Fijians, and Central Americans. Table 1 lists the known and suspected cross-cultural variations of the SP/LD experience.

Table 1.- Cross Cultural Terms and Conditions for Sleep Paralysis

Eskimo/Inupik
Agumangia

Eskimo/Yupik
Ukomiarik

Fiji*
Tarda vakarerevaki

Germany
Doppelganger

Hawaii*
Huaka'I po (warriors, Night Marchers)

Hmong
Dachor

Indonesia
Tindihan

Japan
Kanashibari (totie with metal rope)

Korea
Ka-wi-nulita (scissors pressed)

Mayan/Quiches*
Sak waram (white sleep)

Newfoundland/Europe
Ag Rog (Old Hag) & Nightmare English-speaking version (See Spain's *Pesadilla*)

Philippines
Aswang

Spain (and Latin America)
Pesadilla-duende (little-small weight: also little people)

Thailand
Phi um (ghost covered)

Worl-wide
(?) *Alien abduction cases during sleeping conditions*

Table1, Literature Sources: *Tindihan*, personal communication, Mr. Blasius Winang Asmara; Night Marchers, personal communication,

Mr. Rick Carroll; David Hufford, 1982; Melvin Firestone, 1985 (Bloom and Gelardin, 1976; Ramos 1971; Lemoine and Mounge, 1983; and Foster. 1973); & *personal research: archival, examination of anthropological field notes. To these references, encounters with the "little people" worldwide under sleeping circumstances could be added (see *Microsomatognosia*, next chapter).

Dreaming is mythical. Just like Sigmund Freud, Carl G. Jung, Levi-Strauss, Joseph Campbell, and many others have claimed and tried to proved before me, *that dreaming is an ancient connection to mythical dimension and ancestral past,* I also will end somewhere in this book agreeing with and developing the notion that certain aspects of the dream experience, specifically those that have been explored in ancient shamanism, are still relevant and worth exploring as aids to controlling the negative functions of the SP/LD experiences. *The shamanic interest and approach, as we will see later, emerges naturally from these experiences and need to be weaved into a comprehensive study of the SP/LD phenomena. This shamanic perspective is ultimately rooted in aesthetics, and more precisely, in a psychoecological aesthetics that has served human kind as a mode of connecting with the natural world.* Experiencing SP/LD states forces the exploration of an *ecological unconscious,* naturally, thus I too will need to explore a bit more about the possible outcome of this important connection. It will be argued in subsequent chapters that one healthy outcome of managing the SP/LD experience will land us logically in mythology and in the expression of totemic forms. *Whether or not these totemic intimations and visions belong to a truly pre-human or ancestral human memory and past cannot be proven, but, at the very least, they still could serve as a bridge that can connect the modern and decontextualized mind to a more authentic natural world.*

David Hufford's Conclusion About "The Old Hag" Experience (s)

When attempting to undertake work that includes a summary of the work of many other researchers who have come before one's attempts and interests, it pays to find a succinct set of parameters that may act as a sort of paradigm guiding this rekindled effort. I mentioned earlier in this introduction that reading David Hufford's work gave me an explanation for my own disorder and an impetus to seek and now provide additional information. I would encourage readers to track his book published in 1982, "The Terror That Comes in The Night: An Experience-centered Study of Supernatural Assault Traditions," as a must-read example of a classic reference. From his work, all of it relevant to my discussions in this book, I would like to focus on his concluding remarks about the SP condition and reproduce them verbatim:

1. The phenomena associated with what I have been calling the Old Hag constitute an experience with a complex and stable pattern, which is recognizable and is distinct from other experiences.
2. The experience is found in a variety of cultural settings.
3. The pattern of the experience and its distribution appear independent of the presence of explicit cultural roles models[12].
4. The experience itself has played a significant, though not exclusive, role in the development of numerous traditions of supernatural assault.
5. Cultural factors heavily determine the ways in which the experience is described (or withheld) and interpreted.
6. The distribution of traditions about the experience, such as those involving the Old Hag or the Eskimo

augumangia, has frequently been confounded with the distribution of the experience itself.

7. The frequency with which the experience occurs is surprisingly high, with those who have had at least one recognizable attack representing 15 percent or more of the general population[13].

8. The state in which this experience occurs is probably best described as sleep paralysis with a particular kind of hypnagogic[14] hallucination.

9. Although there may be some connection between the etiology of this experience and narcolepsy, and although certain illnesses could be confused with the experience, the Old Hag experience itself does not indicate the presence of nay serious pathology[15].

10. The contents of this experience cannot be satisfactorily explained on the basis of current knowledge.

As my endnotes convey, I feel, with the exception of his last point, that Hufford's assessment of the Old Hag and other cross-cultural occurrences as descriptions of SP was/is correct. Since Hufford wrote his conclusions, however, more information has been published that is shedding light on this connection and on the psychobiological underpinnings of SP. The last point also necessitates a revalidation of older ancient wisdom or what it is generally referred to as *shamanism*.

To conclude, multiple factors have to be pursued in order to fully understand a culturally and psychologically rich experience, with physiological underpinnings, that can be described by additional medical, and earth scientific methodologies. It is no wonder that, as a default, the individual SP sufferer falls back on the immediate phenomenology of the experience first, trusting the intense subjective reality of the experience, and then seeking confirmation elsewhere, typically, in the many uncanny stories that each culture provides to validate and explain these experiences. As we allude to the mythical and *shamanic* literature we may find that some of these stories and practices may still have relevance today. We will have to find a way to speak about their wisdom and co-opted for our modern purposes.

It is my hope that sufferers and non-sufferers of SP alike, as well as medical/therapy professionals, will find the information in this book revealing of the intricacies of dealing with the impact of dream phenomenology in the psychology of the individual and his/her cultural milieu. Equally, it is my hope that by dealing with the subject in a serious, systematic and scientific manner, as well as presenting personal narratives, and by bringing in classical literary and historical sources (shamanism) much of the misunderstanding and confusion about this uncanny experience, **Bound Lucidity**, will dissipate. At the end of this attempt at elucidation I will be promoting the skill of using SP states to reach other dreamscapes in a controlled fashion in order to achieve mind manifesting and highly creative states of consciousness. *The scientific approach to SP ought not to deter those of us who experience SP routinely from going a step beyond experiencing, intimately and subjectively, these fascinating dreamscapes and potentially positive life-altering modes of being. A balance is being struck here between the scientific explanation of SP as a syndrome, its control in order to appease panic states, and its potential use for creativity and entertainment.*

Methodology

The reader should be alerted to the diverse types of scientific methodology used to arrive at many of the interpretations of the data that will be presented in these pages. Throughout the book there will be reports and examples of quantitative and qualitative methodology. When it comes to my own research, there will be reports of statistical analyses based on correlation data, as well as analyses made using a geomagnetic flux index[16]. Analyses of variance and Fisher least tests were conducted in order to establish a preliminary connection between geomagnetic activity and the likelihood that an SP episode would occur. Additionally, the data is based on longitudinal case studies (ten years), large sample questionnaires, numerous prescribed narratives, and several in-class psychology experiments. The data that Hufford published in his seminal work consists of fieldwork, detailed interviews and polls. The electrophysiological methodology and data from Takeuchi et al and others is described in their studies and referenced in the bibliography. The combined set of studies reported in this book comprises literally thousands of sleep hours and subjects, specifically looking at SP phenomena. I beg the patience of the reader in Chapter One where I present a summary of these endeavors using technical and clinical terms that may slow the pace of some readers.

Notwithstanding the collective suggestive and tantalizing research up to this point, the usual caveat for the need for more research needs to be added. All this evidence is, I am sure, a drop in the proverbial bucket of a possibly larger cannon of studies in the future that could confirm earlier reports; always add new and significant information; specify the genetics, psychochemistry and psychobiology of SP; and construct more inclusive paradigms of the syndrome. Anticipating some remarks in the concluding chapter of this book, many more studies need to address, for example, the commonalities and continuity between SP and other sleep phenomena such as OBE's, ghost encounters, incubi, alien abductions, kundalini, lucid dreaming, and other related phenomenology. It is an exciting time to be involved in the systematic elucidation of Bound Lucidity!

Chapter One

Historical and Scientific Background and Latest Research

"By experience must be understood the entire mental product . . . Hallucinations, delusions, superstitious imaginations, and fallacies of all kinds are experiences, but experiences misunderstood."

C.S. Peirce, *The Concept of God*

A Speculative But Reasonable Historical Background

Most mammals enter REM sleep. The human animal shares the same medullar structures that regulate sleep with the rest of its placental brethren. We the human animal, as a mammal endowed with the capacity for higher reasoning, even infer a dreaming life when we see our sleeping cats and dogs enacting what seem to be daily motor routines and activities. We may not be scientifically certain that the dreaming cat is capturing chickadees in mid flight or the dog tearing pack-rats to fluffs of fur, but I will not, even as a scientist, deny them a complex dream experience. If cats and dogs were not mostly paralyzed during these dreaming experiences, it would be harder to be a pet owner! More importantly, the consensus among scientifically trained and read physical anthropologists and paleontologists are that the human brain has changed little in 150,000 years. This enormous time span that includes five-thousand generations of dreamers and their stories, no doubt many times recounted sitting gathered, around poorly oxygenated fires, inside caves or in compact and narrowly constructed huts; stories told sometimes during psychically/emotionally altered circumstances due to fear, hunger, fasting, religious ritual, or mind-manifesting herbals, will produce, no doubt, uncanny[17] dream life explanations that will endure for generations. If only a small percentage of the entire human population, say 10-16 percent or so, have experienced SP even occasionally, this amounts to a trillion-plus of stories across the ages and continents that deserved and found a cultural explanation and treatment. Additionally, if we can reasonably assume that a smaller percentage of the human population, say up to 3-5 percent, have experienced SP more regularly and intensely since time immemorial, still, this too amounts to a potential wealth of spooky and unsettling round-the-fire conversations about the uncanny that must be accounted for individually and collectively.

What kind of counsel would the elders, listening attentively around an ancient fire, have provided to a young woman of 26, Case "G" one of our subjects, if she had related the following uncanny story to them?

"When I looked up there was this huge beast with its front legs on the end of my bed. It was black and four feet tall. Probably four feet long too. It was muscular—very big. But what I remember the most is its teeth. It had these huge teeth and growled at me. I couldn't move. It came up onto my bed at me and growled and breathed on me. I remember its breath was very heavy. It snarled at me one last time and those teeth came at me—about a foot from my face. I could feel its breath. Then it disappeared. I struggled out of the paralysis fairly quickly and woke up."

What would cross-cultural and ancient traditions that held (hold) sleep and dreaming life to be the bridge connecting the realm of soul to the realm of the living tell the same young woman when she, frequently around these ancient fires while seeking relief for her symptoms, adds components to her dreaming experiences that include real, heartfelt statements such as:

"I could hear a loud buzzing in my ears and it became violently windy . . .

. . . I am beginning to float out of my body . . . I feel my body vibrating . . . do feel the feeling of presence sometimes but usually is just perceive as some invisible thing touching me, or trying to pull me out of my body, and it is not really malevolent—just there . . . one time, and this is actually kind of funny, I 'woke up' and these little people about two feet high dragged me out of bed and onto the floor. It always happens when I am lying on my back . . ."

We can reasonably speculate[18] that depending how tolerant, how familiar these ancient cultures were with this particular set of symptoms, or how determined they were to find practical coping strategies to manage her dream experiences and to prevent these creatures, demons, from affecting the dreamer, her family, the whole kin group or clan, many possible outcomes were likely. The young woman could have been isolated and put through purification rituals, or a special diet may have been prescribed, or different sleeping positions tried. She might have been asked to perform a sacrifice, or to accept blame for an unlucky tribal event, or to apologize to a loved one for secretly or overtly harboring ill feelings toward them. She might have even been thought of as having shamanic potential, thus being taken under the wing of the present shaman for special training to expand and control these faculties. Or worse, she might have been ostracized and exiled or executed for being friendly to dark entities, for consorting with devils. The many folklore traditions, maybe even based on very ancient lore, that specifically address and describe SP, in their own words, survive to this day. The specific names and long-told historical descriptions suggest, at least, a continuity of SP phenomenology and also an attempt to deal with its phenomenology, therapeutically and spiritually. Furthermore, the present era of space travel and impressive visual media that depicts science fictional and science speculative extraterrestrial encounters and wishful-thinking intimations with superior consciousness and intellects, has, in my opinion, given rise to so-called alien abduction stories, that curiously occur in the dark of night, inside private bedrooms, without witnesses, while experiencing paralysis that today can only be reasonably attributed to an unusual type and dynamic form of REM sleep experience (notwithstanding the popularity of a handful of amateur hypnotists and well-intending but unscientific folks who wish so-called alien abduction were true for reasons unclear).

It is true that all manners of demons have their epochs and are in vogue or not depending on what religion and dogma dominates or what degree of medical scientific knowledge exists. Schizophrenia, epileptic seizures, hysteria, the common cold, or simply being cranky for no reason have been 'demon-produced' at one time, only to be later understood as medical conditions, personality disorders, or simply, as being cranky. Presently, with the relatively recent discovery of REM sleep— occasionally referred to as a "third state of being"—by then graduate student, E. Aserinsky[19], and subsequent publication of his data in the year that I was born, 1955, and the advent of volumes of electrophysiological[20] as well as quasi-experimental and correlation data, we too offer an explanation for SP that may finally bring some lasting comfort *to people who really experience these events, are really perturbed by them, and are definitely and greatly impacted by their emotional insinuations.* It is interesting to note, that Aserinsky made his foundational observations, partly, while enlisting the help of his eight-year old as a subject. I believe that our 'demon' and explanation, or some version of it, will endure as long as there is a scientific method or rational system of organizing qualitative dream content data that pursues sleep as a brain state(s), and so long as we make the assumptions I outlined in the Introduction about: the dynamism of sleep stages; the understanding of the preeminent (and sometimes insidious) quality of subjective phenomenology; and finally, the acceptance that cultural lore and context as a dual-edge sword both preserves and taints individual and historical phenomenology. Those of us who practice these principles and are aware of their caveats, and in my case, who also experience SP on a chronic basis, have the duty to ease other dreamers' fears and facilitate the benign forms of the uncanny. In the next section I will hold true to this duty by sharing a brief and restrictive, but I believe inclusive, recent medical and scientific history of efforts to elucidate SP in the last 160 years or so. This systematic description and discovery of sleep behavior and physiology may seem long enough to dispel the misunderstandings that SP sufferers have about their condition. But the reader must also keep in perspective that the characterization, understanding and scientific explication of mental phenomena was plagued, in the west, during the same 160 years by competing ideologies, schools of psychology, philosophy, and diverse methodology. Even today, I frequently hear patient stories of a psychoanalyst, or psychologist, and seldom, a psychiatrist who tries to minimize the biology of the SP experience, or exaggerate some unconscious and un-testable aspect of the sufferer's psychology without addressing the immediate and obvious phenomenology. Regularly, the overwhelmed health provider may have little cross-cultural mental training, much less the time to search through historically based volumes. Therefore, he or she may lack a global demographics perspective and may miss real statistical information about the prevalence of SP. In some situations, prescribing generalist drugs successful in the containment of other sleep disorders is used as a quick fix without trying to address the long term consequences and ramifications of living with SP and perhaps even using its own phenomenology for creative and mind personality aims.

Western Medical History of SP

As we have seen, many cultures have described SP symptomology, but its earliest western, *medical* description appears to be an account by E. Binns in 1842. Binns termed SP a "daymare." Thomas J. Nardi quotes Binns' description (1981) as a patient was falling asleep and experiencing this *daymare* as:

"(The patient was) seized with difficult respiration, extreme dread, and utter incapability of motion or speech . . . [he] could neither move nor cry . . . during all this time . . . [he] was perfectly awake."

Jerome Schneck (1977) also reports an early description for SP in 1876 by S. Weir Mitchell who described sleep paralysis then as "night palsey." However, Schneck gives credit to Wilson (1928) for coining the term "sleep paralysis." For most of the 20th century, SP was written about as a sleep disorder correlated with anxiety and neurosis, that had to be treated psychoanalytically and clinically, or as one of several symptoms that describes narcolepsy [Wilson (1928), Schneck (1948, 1952, 1957, 1960, 1961, 1966, 1969, and 1977), and Hishikawa (1976,1978)]. For example SP was (and is still) mentioned as one of four symptoms associated with narcolepsy, the others being sudden sleep attacks, cataplexy, and hypnagogic hallucinations. Jerome Schneck holds an important place in the modern history of SP research as the person who single-handedly brought its phenomenology to therapeutic circles, and encouraged and mentored others researchers to pursue this investigation. He made an additional and important connection that I will pursue fully in Chapter Two, namely, the observation that one of his patients who experienced sleep paralysis also reported *microsomatognosia*, or experiencing one's body shrinking or reducing in size[21]. *Microsomatognosia* (and *macrosomatognosia*, see footnote) can occur spontaneously and can explain for the accounts of SP experiencers who report little people, or small creatures bedside them or giants looming over them (refer to introduction case story). This skewed perception and hypnogogic hallucination will be used later as an explanation for the so-called alien abduction phenomenon as well.

Moreover, there are many more reports that describe SP in the Americas that are part of folklore studies, anthropological field observations, or recounts by travelers who made a connection to the Old Hag. Basically, the more one digs into the multidisciplinary literature the more SP accounts one finds described, sometimes without the recognition of its global prevalence, that is, simply as a decontextualized local and curious story only. As I have had to augment and strengthen the evidence for my "ring of fire" hypothesis for the SP occurrence, I have interviewed individuals from these cultures, and read folklore accounts of what others would have called "ghost stories."

Researchers who are coming new to SP research and the average reader will be well served by reviewing all this pertinent literature. Even today I review or read articles by other researchers who omit this western history and foundational literature (to the detriment of their studies and interpretations I believe) and imagine that they have discovered SP, or that SP is a uniquely Asian phenomenon that western medical science has not heard of, or, mistakenly, that SP descriptions are not as abundant in other social scientific fields as they are in medical circles. I apologize to the reader for this small peeve and digression.

Clinically speaking, The American Sleep Disorder Association criteria for the diagnosis of SP are: a) the patient's inability to move his/her body (trunk or limbs) at sleep onset or upon awakening; b) brief episodes of partial or complete skeletal muscle paralysis; and c) that these symptoms occur independently from other psychiatric disorders such as hysteria (Takeuchi et al., 2002).

A change in the direction of SP research shifted when authors such as Goode (1962), Everett (1963), Penn (1981), Hufford (1982), Firestone (1985), and Fukuda (1987, 1991, and 1994), began to describe the phenomenon of SP in the context of culture, and other studies followed that estimated: 1) the prevalence of SP in the general population, particular country and ethnicity; b) the prevalence of SP in at-risk populations from a potential sleep depravation perspective (medical students, nurses, college students, air traffic controllers); c) the prevalence of SP looking at subjects' reports of paralysis or subjects' reports of "pressure" on the chest, or both; and d) the prevalence of SP cross-culturally. Table 2 lists most of these studies and the complete citation is referenced in the bibliography.

Table 2. Reported Incidence of SP in Different World Populations While Using Diverse Criteria For Reporting SP

Nationality	No.S's	% Reporting SP	Reference
American medical & nursing students	359	4.7%	Goode, 1962
" " "	52	15.4%	Everett, 1963
Newfoundlanders	76	23%	Hufford, 1970
American medical students	80	16.3%	Penn et al., 1981
African Americans	(?)	39%	Bell et al., 1984
Nigerian medical students	164	26.0%	Ohaeri et al, 1989
Nigerian nursing students	95	44.0%	Ohaeri et al, 1992
Chinese (Hong Kong)	1,020	35.0%Pa*;16%Pr†.	Lee et al., 1998
Japanese	264	22.0%Pa;9%Pr.	" " "
American	202	22.0%Pa;12%Pr.	" " "
Germans and Italians	8,085	6.2%‡	Ohayon et al 1999
International Sample	92	7.6%Pa-only	Conesa, 2002
" " "	92	16.3%Pa&LDs	" " "

Table 2, Notes: *Pa: Paralysis only; **†Pr:** Pressure on the chest; Lifetime prevalence;

- Without any other symptoms; **PC:** personal Communication;
LDs: With lucid dreams. Notice that, generally speaking, the prevalence of SP increases as a function of occupational choice when sleep depravation is suspected to be a factor.

It became clear from these demographic studies (summarized in Table 2) and efforts that SP in the absence of narcolepsy, or Isolated Sleep Paralysis (ISP), was reported frequently by a fairly high percentage in all of these populations. However, and still a challenge for discovery, depending on the criteria employed when asking subjects about their SP experiences (with or without paralysis—pressure in the chest only, report of OBEs or FOPs—feeling-of-presence, reports of incubus, and exclusion of other psychological disorders, etc.) the prevalence of SP in the general population could be as low as 2% or as high as 50%! In my last survey and review of the literature[22] that specifically researches SP and ISP, there were at least fifty references that focus on one or more of the previous aspects of the disorder.

Table 2 then is an unfinished summary of some these reported incidences. Both the casual reader and the SP sufferer may be impressed by the different percentages obtained. As a researcher I suspect that this range waxes and wanes partly because different criteria are selected during the crafting of questionnaires, and secondly, because all these polls are moments in time and samplings of populations that may either underestimate or overestimate the phenomenology of SP in their own memory. So, we should trust these data as much as other reports that use memory of salient, personal events as data. As a humbling example of the fact that anybody can be fooled by the intensity of their own SP experiences, before keeping a precise record of my own SP episodes I overestimated their frequency (see actual figures in Table 3). Other alternative hypotheses might be that the differences obtained in the various samples, assuming that proper standards for questionnaire construction and methodology were used, suggest:

a) *a genetic pattern for SP where same-culture, same-ethnicity groups have locked in a group of SP-responsible genes and thus created a greater probability for as yet described SP genes to concentrate in that particular population or group*

b) *that unique cultural, religious, or ethnic personality or social patterns give rise to different frequencies of reported SP phenomena*

c) *that transient or permanent but socially or familial unique behaviors such as work habits, war-generated circumstances, and other types of stressors affect a given population unduly, to a greater degree; or*

d) *that regionally unique geological or geophysical forces influence brain electrochemistry and therefore psychology, edging up the likelihood for the occurrence of SP in sensitive individuals; or, as one of my research mentors used to say, a combination of any of the above considerations.*

In my mind, these are all scientifically testable hypotheses, and extremely interesting research paths for new generation of sleep/dream scientists. Finally, when it comes to understanding the causes for these incidences of SP, our research is still in diapers.

The Work of Dr. Tomoka Takeuchi

Everyone looks up to a handful of role models in one's profession, and admires the work of these individuals who have left a significant legacy in a given domain and/or are presently defining the next generation of experiments that are said to be foundational. Even though my work has benefited from the collective efforts, findings, and insights of the fifty or so SP influential references alluded to earlier, I keep going back to, obviously, Drs. Jerome Schneck and David Hufford's clinical and scholarly work, respectively, and since the mid-nineties, to the work of the Japanese researcher Dr. Tomoka Takeuchi. Since I have already presented Drs. Schneck and Hufford earlier, and will continue to do so throughout this book, Dr. Takeuchi's contribution to the study of ISP needs to be showcased in this attempt at a history of SP research.

Perhaps because a recognizable traditional description for SP exists in Japan, Kanashibari, it is not surprising that a significant group of researchers from this country have contributed so much to an understanding of SP (and ISP). Takeuchi's work is linked to that of another important and foundational Japanese researcher, Dr. Fukuda. But Takeuchi's work deserves to be highlighted for two important reasons (and that of Fukuda as well). First, because in the orthodoxy of scientific methodology, objective measures of natural phenomena have more weight in establishing cause-and-effect relationships that add credibility to a suspected connection. In the area of dream-sleep research there have been two general paths of discovery: the objective path relying on evolving electrophysiological technology conducted in controlled and aseptic sleep laboratories, and the path of dream recollection studies and analyses, gathered in the real life environment where the dreamer encounters these experiences. As an eclectic researcher, I personally see both pursuits as equally valuable and feel that they compliment each other as well. But going back to Dr. Takeuchi, the second reason his work is so important is because he and his collaborators have been successful in triggering SP episodes in a laboratory setting while using electrophysiological feedback information about sleep stages, thus proving that SP is truly a REM phenomenon. In an earlier study, Takeuchi et al. (1992), by systematically interrupting both NON-REM and REM sleep periods, showed that ISP emerged in REM sleep. Interestingly, and connected with the experience of the emergence of self-awareness during SP episodes, the electrophysiological data showed that indeed, these subjects were awake while in REM sleep. In a more recent study (Takeuchi et al., 2002), thirteen Japanese subjects[23] who had experienced SP spent three consecutive nights in the sleep laboratory of the Tokyo Metropolitan Institute for Neuroscience. Takeuchi and his collaborators were able to obtain eight ISP episodes while interrupting sleep onset REM periods (SOREMPs). Both findings are what health providers, counselors, and the general population need to know about, in my opinion, to begin to understand the intricacies and dynamics of sleep and dreaming, in an attempt to ease the fears of those who report SP. Dr Takeuchi's work suggests simply and elegantly that the SP episodes, at least the ones triggered in a laboratory setting when researchers can actually correlate behavior, narratives and electrophysiology, originate in a physiological state we more or less understand, and equally, in the self-aware creativity of these REM states. By extrapolation, we must assume that SP experiencers in their own homes are dreaming in REM moments as well. Important for a normalization of the SP disorder, Dr. Takeuchi and his staff did not witness the presence of Old Hags, little people, or extraterrestrials running around the laboratory in conjunction with these subjective reports. Nor has anybody else for that matter. Not that some of us did have any doubts, but this means, of course, that it is the individual psychology and/or the culture that predisposes the anticipation or experience of these hypnagogic hallucinations.

A Ten-year Longitudinal Study and Case Study

I experienced my first episode of sleep paralysis concurrent with a so-called out-of-the-body experience (OBE) in 1969.

The indelible experience at an impressionable age of fourteen occurred while in preparation for going to sleep. I remember closing my eyes as if merely resting them, without being even being tired, and opened them only to realize that a rough surface was near my face. This surface, I realized, was the texture of the ceiling in the bedroom I shared with my brothers. Upon realizing this, instinctively, I "turned onto my belly" and I "saw" my (physical) body sleeping about two meters below. The impression of perceiving myself to be "floating" above my sleeping body caused me to awaken in a sudden jolt. The rest of that evening in 1969 was punctuated by several ISP episodes. My account is in no way unusual as first SP experiences go. Subjects frequently mention an OBE experience occurring with their first SP. Several of my subjects have reported very similar first-time experiences. But I find that the following narration, for example, which I received while writing this book from a 16-year old male, Case "MG," is pertinent to my own description:

"Recently, for the first time, I experienced what I think you described as dream paralysis. I awoke from sleeping (well I thought I did) with my face right in front of this plastic spinning coil I have suspended from my fan over my bed in my room. I thought I had awoken and decided to throw myself on my back, onto my bed. I did this, and slowly floated down onto my bed, that scared the hell out of me. Once I landed in my body my nuts (yes my crotch)[24] started to sink intensely into the bed. I had the strangest sensation in my groin, of it just being pulled into the bed, and then I woke up."

Since my first SP episode that evening, and for the following thirty-three years until the present, I have lived with ISP in regular to chronic epochs. *Since that initial experience, I have wrestled with several hairy beings in my own bedroom for nights at a time; been visited by many hags and beauties; been whispered to, shouted at, buzzed, electrified, boomed, and hurt; been touched, pinched, and caressed by phantoms unseen; cried empty screams without anyone hearing them; been assisted by friendly entities who taught me how to move from the paralysis into lucid dreams; meditated in lucid dreams, attaining sublime bliss; been visited by angels; had countless conversations with "elders" who themselves prescribed acts that led to being a healthier and stronger person; cavorted with, been transformed into and played with mostly mountain lions, birds, and deer; and "flown" to places indescribable until flight itself is assumed to be an intrinsic right and property of the body-mind.* Nowadays, for me, SP is hardly frozen panicky immobility, but a sign and signal that announces more interesting phenomena to come; and the lucid dreaming experiences that follow are mostly mind manifesting and creative encounters with the uncanny. But most of you will be even more surprised, I am willing to bet, if I told you that as an agnostic scientist, I still have no opinion about their ultimate reality if there is one, nor do I subscribe to New Age or religious theories (Carlos Castaneda, Robert Monroe, or otherwise) that, supernaturally or metaphysically, account for these experiences. I "simply" call them my uncanny sunset stories, nothing more. They are at the very least, extremely interesting experiences originating in REM dreaming and being fed, I guess, by my unconscious and conscious mental processes.

The result of all these experiences, however, the history and regularity of these events and related dream experiences, coupled by the real need to begin a science of observing and quantifying these regularities prompted several early studies (1988), some of them published since 1995. From these experiences and by learning to cope with SP, the idea of employing ISP as a cue for moving into Lucid Dreaming evolved. As I found out later in my interviews with other experiencers, many subjects who have participated in our polls and have contributed narratives have made similar discoveries, all of us independently of each other. This creative and evolving aspect of the SP experience into creative, lucid and "mobile" states is (was) largely ignored in the SP scholarly, scientific/clinical literature and were not a focus of the seminal and continuing work of Stephen LaBerge (1980; 1995) with Lucid Dreaming techniques. Before exploring these connections in later chapters, I will first share some of the barebones data connected with conducting a long-term recording of the SP experience. These data may be useful to many readers who already keep dream logs and have accumulated SP data as well.

The work (Conesa, 1995; 1997; 2002) of systematically recording nightly dream events began on August 13, 1992 and ended on the same day in 2002[25]. The impetus for conducting these naturalistic observations of dream recollection and logging them systematically came because of a real need in the sleep scientific literature, and specifically in SP research, to gather this type of fully contextualized data. That is, I and other authors [Hall & Van de Castle, 1966; Domhoff, 1969; Cohen, 1974; Gackenback, 1991] felt that realistic and long-term tracking of dream experiences in the context and natural environment of the dreamer, affected by daily life situations, would better describe what actually happens when folks dream in their private lives. The daily frequencies of any dream event were duly recorded according to the methodological guidelines described in Conesa (1995, 1997).

The focus of the study was less about describing dream content (although I recorded these as well), than about accurately taxonomizing and keeping daily frequencies of ISP incidents and other dream events. Choosing to keep track of dream event frequencies, instead of focusing on dream content analysis, made sense in the context of my efforts to quantify the long-term prevalence of SP in a chronic SP sufferer. In contrast to dream content analyses, where dream material can be judged from a subjective and an "outside" perspective, frequencies come closer to an objective evaluation of SP experiences that can then be compared to similar studies without hyperbolic interpretation. Dream content analysis was however an indispensable tool as well, since the SP experience can be recognized by the careful description of its obvious symptomology and phenomenology. In this sense, dream content analyses that focus on a particular class of dreams, or on a particular syndrome such as ISP, looks at a finite set of narratives-as-symptoms that once evaluated, may provide a means for universalizing the experience. In this way, the focusing on a finite set of variables increases both the validity and the reliability of the findings. To be quite honest, I am suspicious of psychoanalytic efforts which converge, without looking at many other psychobiological, mythical dimensions or psychogeographical factors, on a narrow or idiosyncratic diagnosis based on neurotic or psychotic themes that may or may not exist in the dream experience. Anxiety, and thus neurosis, may be simply the symptomatic front of a real fear and uncanny circumstance that it is not self-created. Thus, when a psychoanalytic approach was used to interpret the SP experience, the careful analysts must consider whether it is the lifelong, historical, ontological suffering of the patient with SP that leads to a purported neurosis, a causal factor rather than a symptom to some other neurosis. To be fair, I think it is possible that a person's unique response and adaptational strategies to a real REM bodily paralysis and to his/her hypnogogic hallucinations can provide a window into the psychology of that individual. This is invaluable information for sure, that could be used to chart counseling strategies with the aim of mastering uncanny dreaming.

In short, ISPs, lucid dreams and other dream-related events were recorded on a calendar, usually within 20 to 40 but always within 60 minutes upon awakening. As the experiencer of SP and persons who dream vividly can relate, and unlike the poor memory reported for other more vague dream experiences, the SP experiences in particular are easy to recall, record and keep track of, including, lucid dreams, flying events, FOPs, OBEs, vivid, and extra vivid dream events: they are bizarre dream experiences with a high degree of cognitive saliency.

Spooky Math

This longitudinal, single case dream recollection study, the longest to date, recorded a total of 5,761 dream events over a span of 3,519 nights. All these dream events are broken down by experimental categories in Table 3. During those ten years, the records show that I experienced 228 SP events, or 4% of all these dream events. Furthermore, Table 4 summarizes the frequencies data in percentages and selects five different time epochs or periods of different duration while tracking the prevalence of several dream categories. Interesting is the fact that the percentages and prevalence of ISP changes little during any given selected epoch and still averages to 4% regardless of the epoch chosen. This consistency was not necessarily expected since many aging subjects with chronic SP report the SP incidents declining with age. Further analyses of this data set showed that SP events correlated highly (the second strongest correlation after lucid dreams and flying dreams) with lucid dreams confirming the phenomenological, testimonial reports by others that SP can be used as a launching pad of sorts for experiencing lucid dreams.

Table 3. Raw Frequencies and Percentages Of Dream Events, Types and Categories (N= 5,761 Dream Events)- 3,519 Nights from 8/13/1992 Until 8/13/2002 Excluding 133 Nights (due to travel or illness).

Dream Event	Raw fqs.	%
RD	3,339	58%
VD	839	15%
XV	330	5.7%
SP	228	4%
N(-)	421	7%
SX	306	5.3%
FLY	134	2.3%
LD (ALL)	145	2.5%
LD-S	81	1.4%
LD-I	19	-
LD-C	45	-
OBE	4	-

Table 3, Dream Event Codes (See also Appendix I): * **RD**: Regular (neutral, unmemorable) Dreams; **VD**: Vivid Dreams; **XV**: Extra Vivid Dreams; **SP**: Sleep Paralysis; **N(-)**: Negative Content Dreams; **SX**: Sexual Content Dreams; **FLY**: Flying Dreams; **LD(All)**: Lucid Dreams all types; **LD-S**: Spontaneous Lucid Dreams; **LD-I**: Induced Lucid Dreams; **LD-C**: Controlled Lucid Dreams; **OBE**: Out-of-the-body Experiences. These are exclusive frequencies and dream events are only counted one for each dimension. For example, once defined an extra vivid dream was not counted as a vivid dream nor an incidence of flying was counted as an instance of a vivid dream or of lucid dreaming. Due to errors in printing the number of **XVs** should have been 330.

Table 4. Percentages of Dream Events, Types and Categories from Selected Time Epochs

Epochs	RD	VD	XV	SP	N(-)	SX	FLY	LD
8/'92-8/'95	57	21	-	2.6	10	6	1.2	1.5
8/'92-8/'99	58	17	3.2	4	7.5	5.6	1.6	1.6
1st Five Yrs	58.5	19	1.2	3.8	8.5	5.8	1.4	1.4
Last Five Yrs.	58	11	9.5	4.1	6.4	4.8	3.1	1.4
All Ten Yrs.	58	15	5.7	3.9	7	5.3	2.3	1.4

Table 4, Dream Event Codes (Epochs): RD: Regular (neutral, unmemorable) Dreams; **VD:** Vivid Dreams; **XV:** Extra Vivid Dreams; **SP:** Sleep Paralysis; **N(-):** Negative Content Dreams; **SX:** Sexual Content Dreams; **FLY:** Flying Dreams; **LD(All):** Lucid Dreams all types.

The longitudinal study, albeit a single case study of a chronic sufferer, suggests at least the following:

1. The evidence of other longitudinal case studies, larger samples, and scientific observations undertaken for comparison with the case study presented here may determine whether other chronic sufferers of SP experience the disorder with similar regularity.

2. Given the longevity of the study, other factors, such as geophysical events that are suspected to trigger SPs (see next section), historico-social occurrences, nutritional changes, sleeping habits, etc. can be correlated to the SP events in order to later determine causal factors and important determinants of the episodes.

3. If we take my personal occurrence of SP to be comparable to that of other SP sufferers, then 228 or so incidents of SP in ten years in the life of a naïve, unprepared individual, or a developing impressionable child, could chart a psychological life that departs from the norm in significant ways, both positive and

negative. Assuming an average life expectancy of 75 years today, then this number increases to a possible 1,414 SP experiences!

4. More conservatively, the lifelong frequencies of these experiences in an individual's life, when corrected for a shorter lifespan (Haub, 1995) of 45 years, and beginning SP experiences in adolescence (only 35 years actual SP episodes per sufferer), may be estimated to be actually 684, say 700, ISP episodes for an estimated, historical human population lifespan, instead of my 1,414 SP experiences.

5. In order to understand the potential 'meme[26]' impact of SP stories in the human population and long history, if we multiply by a conservative 2% of a hypothetical total historical human population (Haub, 1995; Keyfitz, 1985-2002) of roughly one hundred billion people, that gives us two billion chronic SP sufferers in the last 100,000 years. The result of this uncanny math provides us with a staggering and speculative total of over a trillion SP events/experiences! Of course, these admittedly speculative numbers underestimate other, larger percentages of the general population that report ISP only occasionally.

6. A rational and scientific approach to understanding SP ought to, in all fairness, begin with the real possibility that, when more than a trillion psyche-impacting SP experiences had the potential of being misinterpreted by the individual or culture as ghost stories, these tales could leave a significant meme-dent on our collective psyches. It is no wonder that the supernatural weighs so heavily on our reasoning as objectively and supernaturally REAL. It is no wonder that the default explanation for SP slides easily into loose New Age descriptions.

Although future longitudinal studies may vary in their presentation of the frequency of ISP in a person's life history, and although other studies and demographics may pinpoint differential frequencies for ISP that are clearly explained in the context of personality, variables, culture, biological conditions, and geophysical or physical parameters, I suspect that none of these new revelations will diminish the established meme-impact that ISP has had or will continue to have in me and other dreamers.

Geophysical Variables

It was, and for the most part still is in mainstream psychology, seen as almost bad taste to pursue, much less put forward hypotheses that hinge on a probable connection between brain physiological events, observed behavior, phenomenology and geophysical events. Specifically, *the question is whether a purely electrochemical gooey mass has co-evolved by interacting with geomagnetic forces, this interaction giving rise to a primed sensitivity resulting in psychological events.*(See Persinger, 1987.)

Relinquishing this opportunity for study prevails in psychology, despite the fact that ecological science has made it into a paradigm that to study an organism without considering its entire evolutionary and ontogenetic context is to miss out on important variables that might explain the behavior being observed. Psychology, as a multifold enterprise that includes both diverse sub-fields of basic research and clinical approaches, has barely taken the evolutionary paradigm to heart, in a profound sense, and in my opinion lags behind biology and medicine due to obsessive scholarly connections to humanistic and sometimes thoroughly anthropocentric multidisciplinary interdependency. As it relates to my theory and research orientations, I embrace evolutionary and ecological paradigms and admit the obvious, of course, that the human organism has co-evolved within a rich geophysical environment that includes many forces. Of course, I also suspect that the human brain, being an electrochemical device, is at least potentially affected by geomagnetic influences. What rational scientist of the 21st century wouldn't? My embracing of a thoroughly ecological orientation has alliances for it hinges on the courageous and scientifically convincing work of Robert Becker and Canadian neuroscientist Michael Persinger, whose work will be highlighted later in the this section.

Notwithstanding that the behavior and psychology we aim to elucidate emanates from a purely electrochemical gooey mass that medical science and its therapy is beginning to treat or influence by electromagnetic means, it may be difficult to think of ways in which the very phenomenology of uncanny dreaming, ISP, might be influenced or triggered by geophysical, ambient events. Conversely, more uncanny than the SP phenomenon itself is the fact that mainstream psychology accepts as its orthodoxy that other physical variables such as temperature, humidity, gravity, pressure on the skin, sound pressure, magnetophosphemes, light waves/particles, etc. impinge the human organism, on the spot, developmentally-historically, and sufficiently so as to create and influence psychological states. All manners of forces seemed weird and unfathomable when unknown. But when it comes to the probability that a changing geomagnetic field, or the many electronic devices, and their field radiations we encounter daily, may have any effect on this purely electrochemical gooey mass, then mainstream psychology shies away from investigation, much less acceptance, with a few notable exceptions.

This is admittedly a defensive way to introduce data which even I call tentative, but it is also a sort of convoluted opportunity to alert the reader not to make more than I am willing to accept from my own observations of a probable association between changes in the ambient geomagnetic field, strength and modulation, and the likelihood that some individuals will experience an SP episode. But as a way of bringing balance to my own tentative explorations, other scientists have tested and cautiously accepted the general hypothesis that there might be a linear relationship (suggesting, with experimental procedures, a causal connection) between changing geomagnetic ambient conditions and behavior and mental health.

Friedman, Becker, and Bachman (1965) found, replicated and wrote about this very relationship for the respected journal *Nature* and concluded that:

"Further investigation must now lie in the direction of longitudinal individual examination as well as in the experimental production and control of geophysical variables to determine a relationship between human behaviors and physical processes."

Their specific interest was in testing whether there was a relationship between periods of intense natural geomagnetic activity and either psychiatric hospital admissions or behavioral disturbances in schizophrenic patients. To both questions and studies focusing on a purported effect cosmic ray, they found such correlation and speculated that:

"In view of the growing body of empirical findings and occasional experimental investigations in the area of the biological effects of magnetic fields, it would seem that the cosmic ray indexes provide a measure of some geomagnetic parameter."

But it was up to Dr. Michael Persinger (1973; 1985a; 1985b; 1987; 1988; 1989; 1994; 1997; 1998; & 1999), who almost single-handedly, experimentally and with correlation studies, investigated across several lines of behavior, physiology and phenomenologies, this connection. His work is so important as it pertains to the connection with the incidence of ISP that it merits a section onto itself as an introduction to my studies.

Dr. Michael Persinger: Geophysical Variables and Paranormal Events

It would be hard to summarize and do justice to Persinger's entire and very creative work and implications to psychology, but at the very least, one or two contributions need to be highlighted before moving to the effects of his work on my geomagnetic research. First, Persinger presented and tested the hypothetical assumption stated earlier to heart and pursued investigations examining a purported connection between mental states and resulting phenomenology being influenced by a host of geophysical variables. More importantly, he showed for the first time that neuropsychological hypotheses were needed and useful in explaining so-called paranormal reports, such as seeing UFOs, ghosts, and even the so-called alien abduction phenomena in connection to neurological liability. Other neuropyschologists have followed this serious line of research; for example, Dr. Peter Brugger looked for causal connections between psychobiological instability and the probability, in some individuals, to experience and report such phenomena; the feeling of presence, FOP.

Dr. Persinger's work has led him to develop experimental devices that mimic or are analogous to earth-strength geomagnetic fields and fluctuation patterns to reproduce, in a laboratory, mystical experiences, to alter memories, to model the sensed presence (a "feeling of presence" or entity) of a stranger in an empty, soundproof room. Specifically, Persinger and his collaborators have shown a correlation between days of quiet, global, geomagnetic activity and archival records of reported paranormal experiences (1985), and between days of decreased geomagnetic activity and archival, reported spontaneous telepathic experiences (1988). Additionally, in a controlled experiment, Michaud and Persinger (1985), while applying an electromagnetic field of 1 gauss strength at a frequency of 5-Hertz for about one minute, were able to affect the memory of their subjects during blinded intervals and trials (with a control, no-field condition). Also, O'Connor and Persinger (1997), again using archival data, reported a high correlation, .90, between Sudden Infant Death Syndrome (SIDS) and an average global geomagnetic activity of 11-15 nT. The same team reported that the incidence of SIDS decreased when the geomagnetic intensity increased to 21-30 nT.

The initial reporting of Persinger's data on geomagnetic activity and psychological and physiological effects gave me the impetus to test his ideas with respect to the incidence of SP. In my mind, the SP phenomenon was a better candidate and model to test a connection with geomagnetic activity, following Persinger's insight and lead, for the following reasons:

1. Unlike the paranormal narratives Persinger et al. had employed, SP experiences were (are) return subjects whose consistence of experience and data could be counted on, trained, experimented with and further replicated.

2. As Hufford had elucidated, the Old Hag/SP phenomenon could also include other instances of so-called paranormal experiences, including, I believe, alien-abduction experiences, FOPs, and OBEs. Thus, an SP experiencer, without a vulnerable or sensitive personality or neurological profile (as in my case), of the sort reported earlier by Peter Brugger or Michael Persinger, would come to the geomagnetic study with fewer and potentially confounding variables to be contended with.

3. SP experiencers, coming from my particular experience, could be taught to compile dream event logs according to some rigorous empirical criteria to maximize data

quality, unlike the archival paranormal data that can be plagued with additional florid subjective elaborations. This cataloguing of dream events develops blindly without knowledge of geomagnetic events. Throughout my studies, I made sure to wait to conduct the analyses (introduced in the next section) retrospectively, episodically every couple of years, thus preventing me from knowing, thus biasing me, the daily geomagnetic changes.

Notwithstanding Persinger's admirable and formidable experimental contributions, I believe my data improves and provides an important confirming model to his, and gives other researchers allied to SP studies data and methodology to test their own questions. The long term data is in the spirit of Friedman's, Becker's, and Bachman's (1965) suggestion that:" *Further investigation must now lie in the direction of longitudinal individual examination.*

The Case for a Probable Geomagnetic Trigger for ISP

The first summary of my SP logs and corresponding changes in the geomagnetic flux was for a 23.5-month period that occurred between August 13, 1992, and July 31 of 1994. In that first report (Conesa, 1995), I was fairly confident that I had confirmed Persinger's hypothesis while looking at the SP phenomenon for this singular case, because an analysis of variance looking at seven days prior and three days after an SP episode showed that two things were happening, as indicated in Figure 1. First, as hypothesized by Persinger, a relative calm period of geomagnetic activity, days—3 and—2 in the same figure, anticipated the SP experience. But, second, and not predicted by Persinger but present in some of the SIDS data he reported, was the fact that the geomagnetic intensity increased abruptly, and the SP experience coincided with the cusp of this increase. My first report also indicated that the Lucid Dreaming experience was even more affected by geomagnetic fluctuations, and shadowed the SP event. Importantly, and acting as a control, geomagnetic activity did not fluctuate significantly, as shown in Figure 1, when random samples of the same geomagnetic index were selected, when an analysis of variance was conducted.

Figure 1: Occurrence of Three Types of Dream Events as a Function of a Changing Geomagnetic Field

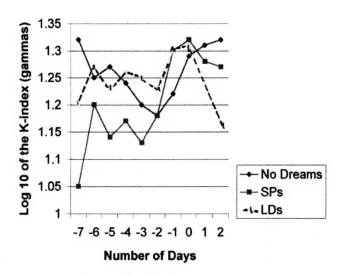

Figure 1.—Sleep paralysis events, SPs, follow abrupt changes— in this figure, rising—in the ambient geomagnetic field. These changes were statistically significant. Additionally, lucid dreaming events, LDs, were also significantly affected by changes in the ambient geomagnetic field. However, no statistically significant changes were found for randomly chosen days were no dreams were reported.

In my second report (Conesa, 1997), using similar methodology and extending the dream recollection and geomagnetic archive into 1,461 days, the results were not as straightforward. Yes, the SP experience, the night event was associated with relatively low geomagnetic activity, but the SP episode was also preceded by an abrupt rise, three days prior, of geomagnetic activity. Specifically, geomagnetic activity declined for three days to the target, SP event night from 18.45 to 13.09nT (significance was at p<.001). This is also a confirmation of Persinger's hypothesis. As a control for these effects, a randomly selected and equal period of time where no dreams were recorded the geomagnetic intensity did not vary: 10.82 nT three days prior and to the randomly selected no-dream target day at, or 10.09nT. I am eager to hear reports of other investigators looking at this possible baseline and non-effect. Additionally, vivid dreams were also recorded in this second study and the incidence of these events paralleled increases in the geomagnetic flux, that is, geomagnetic activity increased for three days to the target, vivid dream event night from 11.00 to 21.25nT (significance was at p<.001). I do not yet know what to make of the connection between an incidence of vivid dreams and a concurrent increase, the sharpest for both studies, of the geomagnetic field. This was simply a post hoc analysis and I did not have a hypothesis to anticipate it nor now have one to explain it. But from my data and the research of others (Lerchl, Honaka, & Reitter, 1991; & Reitter, & Richardson, 1992) *I concluded that the most important variable predicting all these experiences were the abrupt, up or down, changes in global geomagnetic activity.* In short, abrupt changes in the field may be registered at a cellular level, at a high enough level of excitation, in medullar or other dream producing brain areas so as to create phenomenologically felt experiences.

As far as actual probabilities go, my 1997 singular case study data showed that: a) an abrupt change in the global geomagnetic flux of about 12 nT (range 10-14) increased the chance by 41% that more vivid dreams were reported; b) that an abrupt decrease in the geomagnetic flux of about 6 nT (range 4-8 nT) increased by 39% the chance that I would experience an SP episode; and that normal, mundane dreams were reported when the geomagnetic flux stayed constant in the 2-5 nT range.

I had to wait until I had enough data from other subjects to confirm these probabilities and by 2000, after eight years, I had collected 2,972 observations from fifty subjects, including myself. The new numbers showed that:

a)   an SP episode rarely occurred for all of the subjects (probability .10) during days of geomagnetic *maxima*

b)   the probability for the same phenomena increased to .37 if the episode was preceded by at least two days of relatively geomagnetic calm; and

c)   the probability of a reported SP episode increased to .26 for *either abrupt rising or declining global geomagnetic activity.*

Persinger's hypothesis was thus confirmed and revised using the SP experience as a model.

Furthermore, the above results are also in the geomagnetic/physiological functioning range reported by Persinger et al. (1995; 1995b; & 1997); for example, because the occurrence of SIDS increases at the 10-14 nT range but the incidence for this syndrome decreases when the average geomagnetic activity is higher, between 21-30 nT. That is, the average geomagnetic intensity and differential between increased and decreased incidences for SIDS is of about 7 nT (range 11-15 nT). The ranges obtained from the SP/geomagnetic data are between 5-14 nT. We must humbly admit that we simple do not have enough studies, on humans or other animals, to correctly predict the average functioning threshold for geomagnetic activity with respect to the variety of conditions and experiments reported in the last three pages. Persinger speaks of a physiological or (and) psychological functioning geomagnetic threshold occurring beyond 20 nT. This threshold, however, may differ from the physiology and psychological event observed, and from individual to individual depending on their own psychobiological or psychochemical make up.

A final point to consider is that relatively calm geomagnetic days preceding some of these events might act as a physiological baseline, and significant changes to this baseline, up or down, are registered at molecular, cellular, systemic, and finally, phenomenological levels (Lerchl, Honaka, & Reitter, 1991; & Reitter, & Richardson, 1992; Conesa, 1997; and Conesa, 2000). If so, *we do not know whether this physiological baseline is: i) genetically programmed given our co-evolution with these forces; ii) a more recent or relative one being established by the exposure of subjects to the electromagnetic circumstances of their immediate local conditions, including local geology and proximity to household/work sources; iii) or if it is individually, familially determined given unique physiology and chemistry.* I assume that life processes, being more complex than simple, imply that we ought to look at an interactive model that includes at least these three main classes of variables.

On the other hand, the data also indicates that too high of a geomagnetic, ambient intensity adds too much "noise," to use a Signal Detection Theory construct, and the psychobiological system, at least when it relates to dream phenomena, produces no or few dreams. As a scientist, I am not attached to the final revelation or outcome of these hypotheses, only to their testing for the purposes of advancing knowledge of how brain systems may interact with natural and artificial magnetic forces. But I do see and accept the tentative writing on the wall and it reads something like this: *Even small fluctuations in the ambient geomagnetic field, under conditions of abrupt changes up or down, can alter physiology and psychology enough that these changes shape phenomenology, the internal world-view of the subject.*

These changes, as we will see later in the book, may not need to be natural or exclusively geomagnetic in order to have these effects, but establishing baselines and changing these abruptly can be the result of exposure to artificial sources of electromagnetic radiation. In the next chapter in particular, and in others that follow, I will make use of the brief uncanny math and studies highlighted in this chapter, and will attempt to assess their tentative significance with respect to what I refer to as the "average dreamer" in contrast to the many individuals, 2-5% of the population, who report a distinct and bizarre dream phenomenology regularly.

To conclude, the geomagnetic hypothesis is just that, a hypothesis to be tested further in order to answer other mysteries associated with the prevalence of SP, namely, its over-reporting in geophysically unstable regions of the world. But even if colleagues and other readers do not 'buy' the geomagnetic connection, there is enough practical information about ISP in this book that circumvents this premise and focuses on proactive strategies for identifying, predicting, managing and even controlling the SP experience. This chapter was a showcase of numbers and factoids. But numerical facts alone will not give us a complete and satisfactory story of the SP/LD experience. We will do as Galileo did in the words of Ortega y Gasset and:

*"But it happens that reality is not a gift which facts make to man . . . What, on the other hand, did Galileo do? In place of entering the forest of facts as a passive observer and there losing himself, he began by imagining to himself the genesis of movement of thrown bodies, **cuius motus generationem talem constituo. Mobile quoddam super planum horizontale proiectum mente concipio omni***

secluso impedimento." *["I conceive as the work of my own mind a moving object launched above a horizontal plane and freed from any impediment] Only when he has his imaginary reality well in hand does he note the facts, or rather, does he observe what relationship obtains between the facts and the imagined reality."*

CHAPTER TWO

Other Implications of the SP phenomenon

"A knock, the door opens part way, and on the threshold, framed in shadow, stands the figure of the stranger. Neither outside nor in, but in between. Though the stranger knows the name of the one who has opened the door, the one inside does not know who stands in the darkness . . . In this moment between heartbeats, the door is neither fully open nor closed; the choice between fearful rejection or whole-hearted welcome has yet to be made"

Ellen Dooling Draper, *In The Doorway*, Parabola,
The Stranger.

The Average Sleeper

Most people, the average sleeper/dreamer, will never experience the nightly terrifying presence of "the stranger," have to guess his/her intentions, be harassed by his/her touching hands, nor be taken in his/her arms to realms of the uncanny. Perhaps it is better that way, that the entire population does not have immediate and frequent access to the uncanny; otherwise, the trillion or so ghost stories, meme-transported to today, would be so prevalent and unbearable to humanity so as to have prevented many rational developments in the history of mind such as scientific methodology itself. Perhaps cultural adaptations would have been very different, with even more reliance on supernatural or individualist/subjective explanations for natural phenomena. Stephen LaBerge, the scientist who proved to a skeptical dream research orthodoxy the reality of lucid dreaming in 1980, began his seminal and introductory paper with the following statement: "We do not usually question the reality of our dreams until after we have awakened. Nonetheless, exceptions to this generalization sometimes occur when we realize while dreaming that we are dreaming." These two sentences speak to the reality and the chasm that exists between what it is perceived to be a dream and what is not and what is a dream that I AM LIVING and you are not. The "you are not" in this case refers to the "average" sleeper who cannot imagine what a lucid dreamer experiences. When it comes to the SP experience, where dream hallucinations are interlaced with the powerful sensation of immobility and panic, we should add to LaBerger's statement the condition of: now we realize may not even be dreaming at all!

How would the "average sleeper" as a husband, wife, sister, brother, mother or father, reassure their terrified family member who wakes up from a dream or tells them of a lifelong experiencing of SP as in the case of this female of 61 years relating the following (see Appendix III, Case "E"):

"(I) remember the first dream paralysis I had, I was 13 and moved to a new house. I have it all now not as bad . . . pressure on body, cannot move, open eyes, see room but cannot move . . . screaming and wondering if my husband can hear me of if nothing is coming out, trying to move, that when I wake up am exhausted . . . loud humming noise in my head, and I think am going to have a heart attack it's so loud . . . also felt someone putting a pillow on my face and helpless. I think the worse is feeling someone next to me pressing against"

Who can the following case, "JB," consult with after reporting the following (see Appendix III, Case "JB," male, 24)?

"a feeling of being stuck to my bed and I can't move . . . the floating . . . I felt my feet begin to rise, and then my head, but my torso remained on the bed and then my whole body began to tremble with fear and then I was released and I woke up drenched in sweat . . . I felt myself being dragged around the room very, very fast and violently, but the room was empty . . . I sense an evil spirit doing the dragging . . . I heard a male voice and it was coming from the ceiling and it said, 'It's time to play games now.' I strained to get up and finally I did. I got something to drink and went back to sleep but I was very scared. The other voice during another episode was a female voice and it said, 'What are you going to do?' ."

How would family respond upon hearing about these "bad dreams" between sobs and wide-eyed consternation, about what these strange occurrences really feel like? A mother would typically try to console with true compassion, saying something like, "I know it seemed very real to you and that you are very scared, but after all it was only a dream." "A dream? My foot lady!" the child wants to scream, "Tell it to the sinister shadow that repeatedly tries to suffocate me, or pushes hard against my chest!" Knowing the distinction between being awake and dreaming, if he/she is old enough, the child probably realizes that ordinary dreams do not create pain, nor recur with this degree of specificity and collection of symptoms, or with an entity who is always waiting in the dark, motives unknown. The child, more than likely an older dreamer in his/her mid-teens who has read all there is to read about dreams on the internet, probably knows that Dr. LaBerge and other lucid dreamers can change the content of their lucid dreams to whatever they want or wish to create. But our young SP experiencer, unlike the narratives he reads about LD, cannot alter the fact that he hears buzzing sounds and that his body feels electrified before he is even thinking of going to bed; that paralysis will come as surely and quickly as he "falls asleep;" and that neither his screams nor any attempt at shaking himself out of this frozen misery will be witnessed by any family member. Only "the stranger" will be there, as if in a perverted version of the movie "Monsters Inc.," to collect, no doubt, his silent panic or worse, his life's energy.

The "average dreamer" as mom or dad, as spouse or casual lover, needs to understand that *SP is felt with total awareness, with total reality*, because little or no distinction seems to exist between 'inside' or 'outside' perception. This is no "dream" in the usual sense of the word and ordinary experience, nor is it some condition one can easily change, creatively—not at first, at least—when the sufferer does not know what is going on; it is a condition that will affect the dreamer as much or more as anything he/she takes for real in his/her daily life and experiences. The uncanny may even last a lifetime.

If not alone with his/her experience, the teenager may be lucky enough to have a parent, sibling, grandparent, or close relative who has also experienced the SP symptomology and can at least sympathize with the perturbed dreamer. Such is the case in my own family, where my father reported intense dreams, and my own daughter has had SP since she was a small child swearing that, after being paralyzed, she left her room and floated away. I could definitely relate![27] Her SP experiences became so numerous that she established an interminable set of rituals that would keep her awake deep into the night, increasing, as it turned out, the probability that additional SP episodes would occur![28] My oldest son has been diagnosed with a minor form of narcolepsy that includes extreme sleepiness during the day without cataplexy. As a parent who suffers from SP, and thus deeply empathizes with both their difficulties, listening to their descriptions and witnessing their adaptations to bizarre dream worlds or non-ordinary sleep was very worrisome to say the least. I cannot even imagine how a parent who lacks the medical information describing SP deals with the expressed uncanny narrations and descriptions. It must be very frustrating and stressful for both parent and child.

There are things that the spouse, parent, guardian, or significant other can do to mitigate the fear and to reassure the dreamer. *First*, immediate love and reassurance, without devaluing these experiences, goes a long way to gain the confidence of the dreamer. With this love and reassurance information can be shared about dreaming in general or about specific stages if the child or youth can understand it. More importantly, they need to know that they are not alone and that other people experience similar events. *Second*, empirical observations must be initiated that might throw light on the antecedents or triggers of SP for that child or person. Taking (abusing) stimulants like caffeine, high anxiety, extreme physical fatigue, drastic alterations to the normal sleep cycle required for a healthy rest, and significant life changes, may all contribute to SP episodes. If any of these situations exist, they can then be addressed and corrected. *Third*, create a nightly habit and develop a set of simple relaxation rituals that includes massage, soft singing, and deep breathing from the belly area, all with the aim of establishing a regular sleep schedule. More advanced exercises are described in chapters Four and Five that can change the SP experience into lucid dreaming, thus empowering the SP sufferer in her/his dream life. *Fourth*, given how much information is becoming available about the syndrome, the companion will be well-served by gathering the scientific and clinical reports that explain the phenomenon so they can identify further with the experiences of their loved ones. *Fifth*, if despite all these basic home observations and interventions the SP symptoms persist, or become more frequent or intense, then a health provider who understands the SP phenomenon should be sought out. Medication, in my mind, is the last intervention for SP and can only mitigate but never eliminate the underlying causes of SP. As a general rule of thumb, stimulants will increase the probability of SP, whereas anti depressants will reduce it. As an example of the effects of stimulants on the incidence of SP, many subjects have benefited from reducing their caffeine intake four to six hours prior to sleep onset. This reduction in caffeine consumption has the added effect of reducing the level of anxiety originating from another psychic source or daily event. Also, curiously enough, there have been some isolated reports linking the taking of ADHD medication with an increased incidence of SP until the dosage of products such as *Adderal* is reduced or the time taken changed so that it does not precede sleep onset. In terms of reducing the incidence of SP, any medication that reduces REM sleep might help reduce SP episodes. Serotonin reuptake inhibitor medications used to treat depression, for example, *Luvox*, have effectively been used to reduce SP.

Personally, I have not used any medication to control my chronic SP, neither have I sought it for our daughter. It is more important to identify the causes, the chemical, behavioral, or environmental precursors of SP and deal with them so that a better, overhauled life style is achieved than to be dependent on taking medication deal with these experiences symptomatically. My personal preference and perspective is anti-pharmaceutical in this sense, and is consistent with the techniques introduced in chapters Four and Five that explain how the SP phenomenon is transformed from a powerless event to a cognitive signal to pursue creative dreaming.

Ultimately, these are choices that every family has to make on their own with full knowledge of their unique circumstances, and neither I nor anybody else can assume to know enough about this intimate family environment and dynamics. I am the first to acknowledge that if the SP experiencer is very young, and other sleep problems are present such as night terrors or nightmares that make sleep impossible, then a pharmaceutical intervention may be necessary, if only temporarily, until counseling can help manage the situation or until the child grows out of it or learns to otherwise manage it[29]. However, the perspective of the SP dreamer cannot be bypassed for convenience, and their potential lifelong struggle, experimentation and conquering of SP offers an opportunity to advance into states of consciousness that could positively augment anything they do in their chosen life paths. The next section addresses the implications of SP for the person who might eventually come to own the psychological consequences of these experiences.

The SP Experiencer and His/Her Family History of the Occurrence

For the experiencer, "the stranger in the doorway," psychologically speaking, is a challenge, a mystery and even an ambiguous companion that holds important developmental keys. Even when the stranger (FOP) is not a dynamic or frequent element of the SP experience, paralysis itself takes on the role of the stranger insofar as the dreamer's own atonic body, or some "floating" dream version of the physical body, is perceived to be an uncommon and extraordinary experience demanding all mental resources and a cultural explanation. Regardless, the encountering and conquering of the stranger, in his/her own terms and dreamscapes, offers at least four important keys to human development. These are:

1. Connecting the personal and subjective experience to the experiences of other family members so that a "magical" and creative bond might be established
2. The stranger demands attention because he/she stands on a literal and metaphorical threshold of something greater than the fear of encountering him/her there in the darkness
3. The utilization and further development of cognitive skills (like attention and memory) and their further

generalization into potentially all facets of life where hard choices need to be made and where special cognitive skills are required

4. The utilization and further development of courage and its further generalization into potentially all facets of life where hard choices need to be made and new developmental horizons are being traversed

Connecting the personal and subjective experience to the experiences of other family members so that a magical and creative bond might be established. In this sense the stranger in the doorway stands for the gifts, secrets, and promises of older and past generations. These bonds, when narrated in mythology connected or not to the SP experience, psychologically (mystically, spiritually, or communally) connect the new experiencer to the old and wise grandmother or grandfather who also has "the gift." The secret or special intimation between young sufferer and wise practitioner begins an uncanny apprenticeship that, if multiple generations co-inhabit the same home and share a common culture, serves as an important meme transmission vehicle for a collection of, semiotically speaking, a code, or signs important to understanding this culture. The fictional character Harry Potter begins his magical training with a familial remembrance and subsequent connection to the uncanny that it is expressed even when the members of his adopted and dull family stand in the way of this awakening. The magical awakening in Harry's case includes learning that his parents were practitioners as he is becoming and that his destiny lies in embarking on their path with courage. Moreover, non-fictional dream narratives and retelling of the uncanny is an expected daily ritual of the *Senoi* people in Malaya[30] as well as a ritual of other cultures (Inuit). Some gamblers choose their numbers, horses, and dogs on the basis of popular dream interpretation books. By the way, in one of these popular sources, to have a dream that includes "paralysis" is obviously "a bad dream" that predicts financial disaster.

Psychoanalysis, emerges coincidentally with the degeneration and dismantling of traditional Europe and prospers in the United States when a traditional American family is reinventing itself. In both situations the professional, as a surrogate father or mother or new shaman, who encourages transference as a clinical method, listens to and interprets dream as mythology (Freud and Jung) or personal unconscious information as a wise psychoanalyst who has important knowledge of these experiences and can help interpret them.

More pertinent to our present exploration of SP, my own case, cases "S", "G", and "A.J." (Appendix III) and many others all point to a familial experience of SP when other transient or behavioral variables that can account for the phenomenon are accounted for. Like studies in narcolepsy, this familial incidence suggests a gene or gene cluster that gives rise to the syndrome, and as in the case of narcolepsy, this gene or genes may be found. In conjunction with a biological cause, cultural and physical-environmental variables may interact with neurological sensitivities (or cause them) accounting for its prevalence in some families but not others.

The stranger demands attention because he/she stands on a literal and metaphorical threshold of something greater than the fear of encountering him/her there in the darkness. The mere presence of this entity, in an intimate space where and when it was not invited, garnishes self-awareness even more by the process of beginning a devoted and committed cognitive involvement with mystery. Like the proverbial and mythical stories of several cultures, a human, superhuman or forbidding creature stands in the middle of a bridge, before an archway or door, at a river crossing or ferry and demands to know the RIGHT answer to an impossible riddle. If you answer correctly you get the princess but not the lion, or you get to drink from the right vessel, or you get to continue your journey across the bridge unharmed, or maybe even eternal life or nirvana awaits you at the other shore. Appropriate to the closing comments and personal view of the preceding section, and an integral sub-plot in some of these stories, medications[31] can be taken to dull the full impact of these unsavory experiences while standing at the bridge. But the prince who gets drunk on a bridge is bound to be pushed off more easily than when he is alert! Regardless of the choice made, and in connection to the familial experience of SP, it may well be the case that the wise grandmother or grandfather can provide important clues to help solve the dream paralysis riddle the stranger posits that allows the dreamer the possibility of obtaining a gift. The actual gifts are the easier and controlled journeys into lucid dreaming states, stand-alone moments of insight in to problem solving situations, singular epiphanies, or an interactive possibility and further dialogue with the deeper unconscious during uncanny mentations. When the stranger is no longer feared he/she can become an ally to further knowledge.

The utilization and further development of cognitive skills (attention and memory) and their further generalization into potentially all facets of life where hard choices need to be made and where special cognitive skills are required. The hyper-attentional skills, the third key, can grow naturally or be learned and practiced, but basically these amount to maintaining self-awareness and the ability to cognitively interact while in dream states with dream objects, procedures, and familiars. The naturally occurring high degree of self-awareness that spontaneously emerges during an SP episode is a first and crucial step that can be used in conjunction with other cognitive practices, including relying on memory and attention to recall techniques practiced while awake, or to bring back uncanny information from dream realms. Dream experiences are both fleeting and short-lived; therefore, interacting in this realm requires disciplined cognitive manipulation of often taken-for-granted mental skills. This is perhaps one of the most remarkable byproducts of the controlled SP experience: that everyday cognitive abilities can be so enhanced and in their uncanny exercise become sharper. This mental gymnastics is a two-way street, as it was alluded to previously, in that exercises practiced while in wakeful states (medication, concentration, relaxation, mnemonics) also make the controlling of the SP dream realm easier. Stephen LaBerge, correctly so, has suggested a similar value for the controlled practice of lucid dreaming.

The utilization and further development of courage and its further generalization into potentially all facets of life where hard choices need to be made and new developmental horizons are being traversed. The fourth key that the stranger hides is simply the fact that courage and courage alone may assure safe passage beyond this uncanny bridge, or beyond other imagined bridges with the assistance of dream techniques. Specifically, courage is needed while overcoming the paralysis state, in learning how to remain calm in the midst of the experience, and when confronting the stranger himself/herself. In short, mental and psychological fortitude are needed in order to pass the "test" of the stranger, and this more robust mental disposition could be transferable to many other life circumstances, to solving other problems.

The creative potential of all of us, but particularly of artists and scientists, could benefit from this generalized courage and hyper-attentional attitude.

The four keys offered by the encounter with the dream stranger are a single revolving door and interact with each other in ways that invent, reinforce and give sustenance to personal psychology, family, culture, the art of sorcery, science as sorcery, myth, and even religion. A small percentage of the population has been able to infuse the learning of these interactions into human history with good and bad consequences, depending on the perspective taken. From the perspective of this book, with or without the familial influence, and existentially speaking, the

SP experiencer stands alone with his/her gift or curse, poised to do something with it. As in any existential act, I argue that this *uncanny doing* can be willful, rather than prescribed or denied by medication or ignorance, leading to many creative and significant moments that will enrich rather than distress or disappoint the dreamer.

Treatment of SP and Scientific Sleep Research

I have responded to, read about, heard of, and can imagine the reactions of the "average" non-SP sufferer and sleep researcher or clinician when they read the above text or earlier presentations of my conclusions about SP. In general, the reactions and commentary to similar passages in other presentations have been in almost equal amounts of amazement, gratitude, puzzlement, confusion, or dismissal. Sometimes I have known for sure, and on other occasions only guessed, that some of the more negative reactions have come from individuals who, as professional psychiatrists or psychologists, have never experienced SP, much less taken dream states to a level where they become an interactive and functional virtual realm. In some instances, assuming a normal distribution for any position, it is futile to even try describing rainbows to the inhabitants of a world where it never rains or where there is no sunshine at oblique angles.

But in denial or not, imaginative or dull, the non-SP experiencer and professional health provider is nevertheless obligated to supply alternative and diverse courses of medical intervention or behavioral action depending on the needs of the first-time and undiagnosed SP sufferer. A growing body of literature already exists that contributes basic and common sense, and counterintuitive ways of managing SP. This basic information needs to be more widely available and one of the reasons for writing the present book is to be yet another voice in communicating these interventions.

Moreover, and of great importance to the sleep researcher or diagnostician, is the fact that there are several sleep disorders and conditions that occur in tandem with SP—insomnia and sleep apnea, to name two important and common sleep complaints. Insomnia in particular can result as a consequence of consecutive and frequent nightly SP episodes. More relevant to SP experiences is William Dement's discovery of the condition referred to as the REM Rebound Phenomenon (1960, 1966, 1999). The REM Rebound Phenomenon refers to the accumulated physiological need to log REM sleep time, whether normal sleep is deprived willingly or imposed by an occupation, and occurs as soon as an opportunity for rest arises. This condition is relevant to both insomnia and SP to the extent that many surveys tracking the incidence of SP have been done using nursing and medical students who, by virtue of their nightly duties and occupation, are forced to forego normal sleep patterns, report SP in greater frequency, and may be doing so because of the REM Rebound Phenomenon. That is, after reducing a significant number of sleep hours on a nightly basis, or after thirty-six hours of continuous and sleepless work, or drastically shifting to a night-shift (graveyard shift, from 8 PM to 8 AM), the conditions are ripe for rapidly falling to sleep and experiencing SP. Given the above, it is not surprising that sleep paralysis is sometimes referred to as "night shift paralysis" by some researchers (Folkard et al., 1984; and Folkard and Condon, 1987) or that SP occurs as part of combat fatigue (Van Der Hede and Weinberg, 1945) where REM Rebound circumstances are likely.

One of our subjects, a psychiatric nurse in Ireland, adds credence to the medical occupation connection. In her ward, colleagues who work the graveyard shift frequently report SP, specifically around 4 AM. This morning hour turns out to be their first opportunity to rest, coinciding with a break, after five hours of sleep postponement. This time frame, it seems to me, is congruent with REM rebound effects possibly contributing to SP. Additionally, a second nurse contributor to our study reports that she began experiencing SP about thirty years ago, coinciding with a twenty-eight year career in nursing. These specific job-related SP experiences have long been recognized in the hospital occupational milieu and have been termed "night nurses' complaint." In conjunction with sleep deprivation in general, it is now known that driving accidents involving a lack of sleep may be more numerous than accidents caused by drunk driving (REF). To this I can add the experience of Micro REM moments that insert themselves in to consciousness and may not be noticed by a driver but which nevertheless render him/her physiologically in a sleep state. Incidentally, I remember driving with little sleep from Eureka (California) to Minneapolis, from Chicago to Seattle, and from Toledo (Ohio) to Miami, and awakening on the road only to find a big truck looming too close to my car, or worse, after many hours on the road, seeing to my horror and amusement strange creatures crossing the road—hairy giants or little people. I blamed such sightings on bad Wyoming or Ohio so-called coffee, but in retrospect, with the literature that I have now read and understood, it is very possible that an SP sensitive individual like myself was experiencing micro REM episodes or was so sleep deprived that I was REM rebounding. I take this to be the most reasonable explanation because although I and others can attest to the watery quality of Wyoming or Ohio coffee, nowhere have I read about the exotic fauna encountered on their roads, at night, in the middle of the night; when the uncanny is projected from within onto the dimly illuminated road screen.

Fewer, but significant nevertheless, are the subject reports of individuals who have been diagnosed with sleep apnea and also report SP. The few cases that I know of deserve mentioning because they involved a diagnosis of sleep apnea *as a result of* the subject relating SP symptomology. In one of these cases, although the patient received treatment for her sleep apnea condition, the sleep diagnostician ignored her second set of complaints that persisted even though a semi-successful intervention was found for her sleep apnea. With so very few case studies it is only a matter of speculation, but part of the classical SP experience in many subjects includes a reported feeling of suffocation and the inability to breathe. It would not be difficult to infer that SP might be confounded, admittedly in a handful of cases, with sleep apnea in such a way that SP becomes the very diagnostic and symptom that makes sleep apnea known.

These medical connections cannot be ignored if patients are to be treated from a holistic and ecological perspective. But beyond the possible confounds or interactive potential of SP is the complexity of the awake-sleep continuum itself. James Austin, while revisiting the literature and his notes on his remarkable work Zen and the Brain (1999), says that a long and dynamic continuum exists between and within the cycles and stages of sleep, alertness and wakefulness, or while in meditation. Depending on what research he quotes, there can be from as few as three to as many as dozens of discrete and discernable consciousness states. This very complexity of diverse consciousness states makes the work of the sleep diagnostician more daunting when several of these states present themselves in unison, or occur so closely together that they give rise to confounded phenomenology. Early approaches to understanding sleep and its disorders underestimated this complexity, and oversimplified treatments. It is commendable that authors like Austin (1999) take on the enormous challenge of placing conscious phenomenology, sought after or naturally achieved, along these more complex continua.

But this ecological approach does not easily or necessarily translates into testable methodology inside the sleep laboratory, or into 'efficient' and outcome based clinical services. In an era of health delivery and services oriented toward profit-cost-benefit considerations, the single-cause, efficient and exculpatory illness management is the norm. When does the mental health provider, barraged with mountains of must-fill-out state forms, have the time to approach an SP related event from a dynamic and fully contextualized perspective?

In SP/LD research, a fully contextualized experience includes an exploration of the role that SP/LD plays in the study of consciousness. This very approach takes SP/LD studies beyond its classification as an odd syndrome with possible mental disturbances to the area consciousness theorizing. The next section proposes a possible link to a particular area of consciousness studies that elevate the role of the thalamus in the generation and maintenance of conscious states and as the neurological strata to look for the genesis of the SP/LD experiences.

Sleep Paralysis (and LD) in Understanding Consciousness with Self-Awareness

Although no one has explained how it is that SP/LD experiencers acquire self-awareness and consciousness during these uncanny dream events, there is mounting evidence to suggest that researchers should look at the thalamus in particular, a tennis ball-sized structure centrally located in the middle of the human brain, for answers. Specifically, Baars, Newman, and Taylor (1998) have proposed the role of the Intra-Laminar Nuclei (ILN) of the thalamus as the neuronal agency mediating consciousness. Their proposal for this structure as the basis of consciousness is based partly on the fact that disrupting this system eliminates consciousness and that it generates, in conjunction with other thalamic systems, a 40 Hertz "binding" neuronal firing associated with awake and alert states (Llinás and Ribary, 1993; Newman, 1995). As these researchers have argued, cortical functioning depends on the thalamus for its activation and sustained operation, making it a source of consciousness, not merely a subsidiary agency.

As Baars argues, consciousness is not eliminated by disruption of other cerebral centers except the medulla. Medullar systems themselves are also involved in arousal, dreaming, and sleep. Then, it seems that SP and LD states present a unique opportunity to test the purported role of these systems insofar that SP/LD events mimic the activity of thalamic systems during waking reality. Important to this exploration is the fact that there is an intimate connection between the ILN and frontal lobe and motor cortex areas (Austin, 1999). In SP/LD states there is AWARENESS of paralysis and a META-awareness of an individual self who is paralyzed. It seems to me that proponents of the thalamic theory of consciousness can falsify their proposal by looking at what happens during SP/LD events.

As the sequences leading to SP/LD in Chapter Five suggests, the phenomenology of SP/LD dreaming can at least suggest how attention is being deployed all-of-a-sudden in the brain of these uncanny dreamers. One common experience during LD is finding oneself with full self-awareness in a dream with the ability, albeit limited by wakeful experience standards, to engage in a virtual environment.

Furthermore, we can consider the analogy that the thalamus, and the ILN in particular, are akin to a traffic cop in the middle of a busy intersection and roundabout. All manner of vehicles, traveling at different speeds and requiring different times to go around the roundabout, stand for the multiple sensory, perceptual, and motor signals processed by the thalamus on their way from and to sensory and cortical way stations. For our analogy to work, given present theories of consciousness, the traffic cop is not merely directing traffic, he/she is both a signaling agency and the conscious hub and energizing agency of all movement. But it is not known in consciousness studies whether the 'cop' acquires consciousness because it must keep track of multiple modalities and needs to integrate and generate a meta-map of its functions, or because it has evolved possessing this intrinsic sense of self-hood, or because the entire cerebral ensemble, pulsating at a unique frequency, generates a distributed and epiphenomenological consciousness.

Regardless, this thalamus cop must take coffee breaks or visit his/her family sometimes and then sleep without consciousness 'happens.' Without making a novel out of this character, let's assume the traffic cop and thalamus collapses of fatigue on the spot, on its high and lofty parapet. Sensory, perceptual and motor traffic also quiet down. Let's assume further that the cop, all-of-a-sudden, "wakes up" in the middle of the night in his/her parapet from a surge of exhilaration left over from a busy and worried day. Certainly, as in the case of the SP/LD experience, he/she might be confused to find out that he/she is awake when there is little or no traffic to direct; moving his/her hands and arms makes no sense.

This very fact is paralyzing! He/she tries to move his/her arms but they are useless. He/she can look around, know himself/herself to be standing on a parapet, and can maybe even leave the parapet altogether and no one would notice.

SP/LD experiencers are in the same situation as the traffic cop whether or not the thalamus turns out to be the cohesive force and conscious energy behind our peculiar state. But the thalamus would be the obvious place to start looking for our wandering lost souls.

Sociocultural and Folkloric: Alien abductions as Birth Memories and SP

A fully contextualized approach to anything may be, realistically, a pie in the sky proposition. Still, most sleep researchers and technicians engaged in electro-encephalo-gramic (EEG) technology and research are trained to interpret REM sleep as, Austin's reference of Llinás and Pare (1991) says, "an active brain in a paralyzed body." This bit of knowledge should already close the gap between what we think of consciousness when awake and some other type of consciousness, usually an altered or alternate (and lesser) form of consciousness not deserving much debate in the Philosophy of Science literature. That is, this bit of wisdom should be enough to begin a phenomenological unveiling that intersects the so-called electrophysiological data with the cultural lore. Because this book is partly an attempt at de-singularizing complexity, semiotically speaking, we need to continue knitting, so to speak, an ecologically richer fabric of knowledge that extends from the individual experience, through the necessity of singularization in scientific enterprises to the cultural lore. We are obligated to do so even though the proverbial tapestry may look a bit patchy and modest looking at first. We can add another color-thread to our patchwork analysis from classical psychology, from the much-maligned study of *psychological archetypes*. This detour may be useful in exploring across these levels in a *pansemiotic*, or if others prefer, *transemiotic* journey.

There is no question in my mind that archetypes are psychologically real entities and that these are capable of influencing cognitive processes or even of directly affecting dimensions of personality, functionally speaking, so as to change behavior. But where do these archetypes come from? Are these genetic in origin as Carl Jung supposes, learned and internalized from cultural heroic or phantasmagoric theme memes, or simply the expressions of hidden and latent personality propensities that have not had a turn in expressing themselves because environmental triggers do not yet exist for their timely deployment?

Rather than answering these questions rhetorically, I will offer another origin for archetypes rooted in the mutualistic relationship between consciousness states, when awake or while sleeping, and the necessity for heuristics during problem solving in real life situations. Archetypes in this sense are guidelines for action, heuristics, for problem solving. If when problem solving we use both conscious and unconscious creative processes to arrive at a solution, then the awake-sleep continuum is potentially traversed in its entirety until we have something: an answer that makes sense. These answers can come from dreams. But the dream content is itself influenced by the events and situations that transpire during the wakeful states (see Lucy Gillis' and my LD excerpts in the next chapter). However, dream story line is of a different sort: often fractionalized, pithy, emotional, in a state of flux, simplistic, and maybe even driven by quick fluctuating cerebral right hemisphere attentional strategies.

The result of this very unique approach to thinking necessitates a different and summed-up language than the one that often takes the form of an archetype. To illustrate, early on in our professional or academic careers we are impressed by a certain mentor or teacher and while interacting with this admirable role model we acquire and internalize many of his/her personality traits, ideals, or mannerisms. These traits, if additionally tied to existing stereotypical societal roles (mentor-protégée), are insidious enough to make a significant dent in a developmentally young, impressionable and eager mind. While consciously identifying with this person or not, these meme traces are the creative ingredients for an archetype. In order for this example to be relevant and widespread one should recognize that both positive and negative role models could influence equally the developing psyche. Additionally, one must recognize that many of these roles are repeated across cultures, thus acquiring universality (Earth Mother, the maleficent joker, the trickster, the wise old man/woman, the devil/shadow, the teacher, the hero, the destroyer, etc.). Recently, while in a lucid dream, I dreamed about my graduate school mentor, at a time when I was second-guessing certain professional and life choices. In the dream, my mentor appeared not in his familiar human or academic forms, but already *archetyped*, after fifteen years or so of absence, generalized to a dream entity who extended his wisdom far beyond the topics of my graduate school problem solving dilemmas. Physically, the dream image was elevated to a demi-god stature for he appeared dressed in a toga, and adopted a consistently gentile and patient attitude.

Thus, associated with the ambiguity of the stranger, is the possibility of many archetypes. The trauma of SP and accompanying hallucinations may elicit even very distant memories in some sensitive individuals. In fact it has been proposed that the alien-abduction phenomena is parsimoniously explained if we assume that some individuals are remembering actual birth experiences.

An Alien-Abduction Story In The Making

The following narrative is a hypothesis based on what Freud discussed in the context of **Hypermnesic Dreams**[32], that is, that ontogenetically true information, which has been processed in the past by an individual, resurfaces in a memorable dream. Although several ideas that Freud proposed with respect to dreams in connection to personality diagnosis may be untestable and irrelevant to the example that follows, the opening of his *The Interpretation of Dreams*, reports of a phenomenologicaly accessible type of dreams, *Hypermnesic Dreams*, where personally-historically true information remained hidden for many years before resurfacing again. The following narrative considers so-called alien abduction reports from this perspective and suggests that this so-called abduction cases as extreme and traumatic forms of *Hypermnesic Dream* experiences which utilizes birth memories as past information and unites an unusually creative and sensitive mind with and an SP event.

A neonate, born with limited sight, is mistreated by a rough team of uniformly colored hospital staff—the grays, the blues, and the greens—who wear masks or strange goggles. These goggles, or even the bare eyes of the medical staff, look to the fuzzy visual world of the neonate, like enormous dark patches. These "aliens" probe the infant in private places and extract fluid samples from different parts of the body. These "aliens" insert probes in anal and oral areas and shamelessly handle and investigate genitalia. They inflict additional pain on an already traumatic experience. Most importantly, and part of the making of a complex context for this developing memory that might be revisited years later, the neonate is whisked and lifted into the air as if by magic, levitating in unseen hands and arms. The neonate cannot control musculature and, paralyzed, not being able to avert or escape any of these insults, is utterly helpless. The infant, probably the most sensitive organism that exists, is pushed away from a cozy, wet, protected and warm place only to find itself surrounded by expressionless beings. To add more ambiguity to the scene, an ambiguity that might even persist in later stories, these beings also caress and touch his/her body producing sensually pleasing experiences never before felt.

The strangely illuminated and aseptic room, inhabited by the "tall" and "shorter" beings, is filled with strange higher frequency sounds that the newborn has never encountered. Buzzing, beeps, drilling, laughter, and a language that is not understood yet, muffled behind tight masks, adds a soundtrack to this unearthly movie.

For the next few days or even weeks, before the infant can recognize patterns, self, mother, the "aliens" come and go as if by magic[33] and they repeat some of the same insults insuring that a certain memory will be permanent. The infant, lacking even the most primitive conceptual categories, must either accept these events at face value, or be forced to create schemas to categorize all these happenings.

The infant is placed on cold tables, in the company of other "kidnapped" babies, themselves confused, helpless and crying. The mother, being the only safety anchor and source of happiness, is instrumental in helping the infant forget these assaults, and in time they seem to forget until one day . . .

. . . the same child, an impressionable child, now a teenager or an adult, experiences his/her first SP event. Then, it is possible that the paralysis, the absolute terror, and the deprivation bring forth a memory context long forgotten (that should be forgotten!). The mostly internal processing of information characteristic of REM sleep searches memory fragments until it recreates the closest experiential context for the present paralysis, namely a situation long ago where an infant lacked motor control, vision was imperfect and blurred, and its body seemed to levitate about only to find itself placed in a crib limited to viewing a singular but crisp percept or restricted field-angle of vision. At the same time, strange sounds are remembered or juxtaposed with other sounds occurring in the sleeper's bedroom.

Add to this hypothetical scenario the memory of a first cat sleeping on the baby's body and the infant being unable to move away from it or make it go away, in fact, continue to add probable and likely scenarios of the many situations that these sensitive babies can and do experience and it is not hard to imagine that at least some of these sensations and perceptions will have an enduring impact provided a similar memory context is recreated in the future.

I am not suggesting here that every so-called alien abduction case connected with an SP experience can be explained in terms of the preceding scenario. But, the principle of parsimony suggests that we begin here and not in outer space to look for root causes. Other authors have suggested the connection between the so-called alien abduction cases and sleep paralysis. For example, Susan Blackmore (1998) has examined this link[34]. But what I am suggesting here is a re-examination of Freud's idea of *Hypermnesic Dreams* and its relevance, if any, to the sleep paralysis/so-called alien abduction phenomenon as birth experiences remembered and distorted into a palpable fantasy.

To reiterate, the experience of "The Stranger" then could also be a memory cluster or memories reinterpreted to fit the present condition that is also uncanny and new. Now enter the biased hypnotist with a flair for writing popular books; enter an understandable and unconscious or voluntary complicity between individuals to play along with the hypnotist and not only are these experiences validated but they are now permanently fixed as the only possible explanation of the uncanny[35].

It is understandable that both experiencers and biased hypnotists are mystified by and drawn to exotic extraterrestrial stories in order to answer the real and bizarre experiences of SP when they lack (or don't care to learn more about) a thorough understanding of the complexities of sleep physiology and phenomenology. On one level, one can understand and forgive this stubbornness as a primal orientation of the human mind to try to explain the bizarre by whatever means necessary no matter how absurd these explanations may be. There might even be an unknown, built-in problem solving heuristic—we'll call it, for a lack of its existence or a proper term, the Symmetry Heuristic, e.g., "fight fire with fire"—as part of our human mind that follows the rule: the more strange and bizarre an experience seems to be, the more bizarre an explanation I need to understand it. On another level, if several of us believe the incredible story then we feel less alone and, as a matter of social reinforcement, are likely to continue believing it.

It is, however, unforgivable that scientifically trained mental health professionals would fan the flames of such fantasy for reasons unknown.

To summarize this chapter, the reader has been exposed to an uncanny ambiguity, namely that SP/LD experiences are a real psychological experience, or more real than any experience that is accepted phenomenologycally, and that these realities lend themselves to different interpretation outcomes: but always in the context of a predictable set of symptoms. Therefore, these experiences are capable of impacting the human psyche absolutely, irrevocably, periodically, and to such a degree that individuals are forced to take stock of their sanity. Given a possible psychologically vulnerable state, and given specific cultural conditions that may exist, individuals who routinely experience SP and LD with accompanying phenomenology exist in at least two worlds.

But in Bound Lucidity, and adding to further ambiguity, "The Stranger" is also the dreamer ready to commence on a journey of discovery, ready to receive wisdom from landscapes created and controlled within. There is no way around the ambiguity of the stranger and we must be ready to face all of its manifestations and decide for ourselves, which one is more healthy and conducive to well-being and further growth.

The ambiguity and potential psychological mayhem delivered by the stranger has been recognized even in times when superstition was prevalent. Specifically, the resolution of ambiguity for any given outcome, positive or negative, is described in the psychedelic, mind-manifesting literature as being influenced by an "experiential set" of both psychological and environmental circumstances. Michael Harner (1981) quotes a fairly lengthy report by a contemporary observer (Ciruelo, 1628) describing the behavior of witches who have anointed their bodies with hallucinogens in order to induce shamanic flights. It is interesting to me that a voice immersed in an era that sees the supernatural as real is sometimes removed enough from this influence to appreciate the complexity and reality of what he observes, real or imagined:

"Witches, male and female, who have packed with the devil, anointing themselves with certain unguents and reciting certain

words, are carried by night through the air to distant lands to do certain black magic. This illusion occurs in two ways. Sometimes the devil really carries them to other houses and places, and what the see and do and say there really happens as they report it. At other times they do not leave their houses, but the devil enters them and deprives them of sense and they fall as dead and cold. And he represents to their fancies that they go to other houses and places and do and see and say such and such things. But nothing of this is true, though they think it to be, and though they relate many things of what passes there."

The *stranger* is trickster the coyote ready to give and to take away at a moment's notice. The *stranger* is a shape shifter depending on psychological or cultural expectation. Accepting a Freudian interpretation again, as impressionable infants and children, mnemonic foundations were laid and so were the seeds and themes for mythical thinking. The alien abduction experience may be, ironically, the least mythical and more real of all the tales because it is grounded in a hospital experience, even though present in the adult, it may be camouflaged as a modern science fiction witch story.

No one can prove that aliens do not visit dreamers as part of some sinister (or edifying and benign; *more ambiguity*) plan to reseed a dying extraterrestrial race. I can only hint here at the probability that the creative power of an already mythical mind, situated now in the middle of the SP/LD experience and not knowing it as such, is capable of manufacturing many stories for defense, comprehension and social adaptation. But these images are persistent in our mythos, reconstructed by a mind prone to *dream*.

To summarize, "The Stranger" represents an open-ended experiential condition that can easily accommodate the internal psychological ongoings of the individual, his/her mind-set, including his/her fears, insecurities and wishes. Additionally, "The Stranger" can be made out to be, provided that a similar memory context exists, the extraordinary images, sounds and sensations once experienced during birth. As I will argue in Chapter Three, these reminiscences, in addition to preserving quite a bit from their original set of sensory data, can be further *archetyped* to represent mythology or important universal personalities (The Old Hag, The Wise Old Man, The Wise Old Woman, The Devil, The Little Devils, Seduction, Hairy Beasts, Angels, etc.).

CHAPTER THREE

Lucid Dreaming and Sleep Paralysis

> *"If you try to listen to every sound in the jungle, what do you hear? You hear more than land animals, water animals, animals of the air . . . more than anything else, one hears the sounds of the steps of animals we have been before we were human, the sound of the steps of stones and of plants and of things that human beings have previously been. And also what we have heard before, all that you can hear at night in the jungle . . . you also hear what you will listen to in the future, what you anticipate, in the middle of the night in the jungle, in the jungle that sounds in the middle of the night."*

Cesar Calvo, The Three Halves of Ino Moxo.

SP and LD

In earlier chapters I defined LD, wrote about the co-occurrence of SP and LD, and argued, more specifically, that SP can be used (is naturally used by SP experiencers without training or suggestion) as a natural cueing and signal to achieve LD states. In Chapter Five I will give a detailed account of a comprehensive system of cognitive and behavioral manipulations, Sleep Paralysis Signaling, or *SPS*, and explain the rationale behind its use above other methodology that has been proposed to induce lucid dreaming states[36]. But before discussing these techniques I shall devote this chapter to addressing the phenomenology of lucid dreaming from another paradigm, that of Aesthetics.

The reason for taking this perspective is that as one tracks seminal literature about LD from the late 19th century to the publication of LaBerge's (1980) decisive empirical work on LD, one notices a thematic pendulum swinging from a supernatural or surreal description of LD states to more scientific treatises and back again to New Age interests and novel technology. Personally, I don't view these movements and discoveries as contradictory or exclusive to the extent that dreaming belongs equally to the private and internal subjectivity of the dreamer, to a shamanic journey rooted in ancestral practices, to commerce, and to the eye of scientific interest. The pursuit of knowledge may take a cyclical form but wisdom and synthesis come from recognizing the existence of these cycles.

But a major paradigm, Aesthetics, has not been written about enough in recent times. Aesthetics embraces all the swings that the pendulum might move into, so therefore, it emphasizes and adds to all these enterprises. It is unfortunate that both present-day mainstream psychiatry and psychological science seem to have dismissed Freud and his *Interpretation of Dreams*, and seem not to be aware of continued literary uses for his ideas that may be relevant and helpful to SP and LD experiencers. In the absence of these sources, we might not have seen an important semiotic characterization of the SP and LD experiences as useful and creative psychological engines in present or ancient times.

Notwithstanding LaBerge's relatively more recent focusing on the creative aspects of LD, the serious study of Aesthetics in literature or philosophy, a more traditional enquiry, brings rigorous analysis, a wealth of sources, and a respect for the mythical aspects of dreaming. The Aesthetics perspective is capable of transcending the supernatural and the scientific points of view to the extent that it reminds us again and again that dreams and dreaming are part of a larger, semiotically complex, and creative realm of metaphorical interpretation of existence, at the cross-roads between discursive and non-discursive expressions or experiences[37].

To put it differently, to the extent that uncanny dreams belong to a unique and special cognitive-experiential realm, or are experienced intensely and routinely by only a handful of humanity, or easily participate in or are part of a larger human mythos, then they are ecologically real experiences capable of powerful psychological transformation that must be understood at their experiential roots by means of their own symbolism and *doings*. This continues to be our work borrowing whenever it is appropriate from the scholastic tradition of Freud and Jung but with a renewed and intense focus on the SP/LD experience.

In this sense the sleep paralysis experiencer and the lucid dreamer, in their experiences and attempts at narrating their dream worlds and visions, are poets. They are sorcerer-poets of the *uncanny* in a similar way as Ino Moxo's opening quote above describing a rich juxtaposition of sensorial sources, objectively external experiences, and the ecology within. Whether pure objectivism likes it or not, humans reach a fuller sense of being by understanding and drawing from this juxtaposition.

Both Sigmund Freud and Carl Jung recognized this and their efforts represent the influence of this aesthetic tradition in the later incorporation of psychoanalysis into literature and philosophy. This third paradigm that speaks to and reflects on dream consciousness is as analytically rigorous as laboratory objective methodology and does not omit non-scientific literary sources. The next section will be a reminder and further exploration of this influential perspective as a way of emphasizing the creative properties of dreaming. In the spirit of full disclosure, the pendulum and study of SP and LD experiences in my case swings two ways—one moving toward the scientific understanding of these experiences and one admitting to and rejoicing in their contribution to my human growth. It is my hope that at least some of the readers of this text will benefit from my brief excursion and reminder of the role of Aesthetics as an alternative position of the creative possibilities of SP and LD states.

Equally important, and as a way of illustrating the creative and psychologically meaningful power of these experiences, the reader will have an opportunity to read about the lucid dreaming experiences of Lucy Gillis, producer and co-editor of "The Lucid Dream Exchange" journal and web page[38]. In addition to being a lucid dreamer herself and being responsible for co-creating an important informational forum for the explication and continued discovery of LD techniques, Ms. Gillis' narratives, in her own words, represents a positive and canonical journey of lucid dreaming and the role of SP in these events. I am very grateful to Ms. Gillis for sharing her first-hand LD experiences and her ideas about OBEs, including her scientifically testable, I believe, hypotheses (Out-of-Phase Dual Awareness) about a possible explanation for some types of SP experiences. It is important to me to present her experiences, thoughts, and ideas as she wrote them so I would not attempt to interpret her own perspective. Her words stand alone as a powerful and clear statement for these experiences. Also, and at the end of this chapter, I have included a personal example of LD that speaks to the mythic, poetic, and perhaps even prophetic qualities of the SP and LD experiences. I have shared this particular story in Lucy Gillis' "The Lucid Dream Exchange" journal and forum.

Mythic Consciousness

It is understandable that SP and LD experiencers alike, frequently finding ourselves at the experiential threshold of the uncanny, seek wisdom beyond the confines and limited narratives—usually toward the dysfunctional or the perplexed—of medical science. These nocturnal experiences are as mysterious and open-ended as the sensorial experiences described in Ino Moxo's rich native Amawacan language and experience. In the opening quote, Ino Moxo capitalizes on his description of a hallucinatory state—the fear, discomfort, and uncertainty coming from a barrage of potential new and internally generated sensorial experiences and meanings lurking "in the jungle in the middle of the night." For some of us, the forced experiences of sitting alone in the dreamy "jungle," without the skills needed to understand its secrets or survive them, can be, of course, a metaphor for our uncanny situation: a multitude of strangers and strange things await us, many coming from within ourselves, from a deep unconscious reservoir, even from an "ecological unconscious"[39]. Sorcery and Shamanism, as we will see in the next chapter, are the oldest sciences that began to make sense of these ancient experiences and may have a lot in common with modern empirical methodology, with the added bonus of preserving the mythical and practical dimensions of SP and LD phenomenology. Within the newer western tradition and its philosophical and empirical methodology, the scholarly study of mythology or of aesthetics may also contribute to this exploration and preparation for the uncanny. Specifically, semiotic studies of meaning, when embedded in poetic legends and ancient narratives, may offer a window and respite that enlighten, diagnose, or prescribe new frameworks for assimilating and accommodating the rich sources of images and archaic motifs that are often revealed in these uncanny explorations.

To reiterate, between the supernatural and the natural there is an third perspective of thinking about SP and LD and this perspective comes from aesthetics. More importantly, philosophical inquiries into aesthetics (in collaboration with other fields such as psycho-aesthetics), specifically into an understanding of poetry as an art form, have already charted a path, created a vocabulary, and have analyzed the nature of dreams, poetic creativity and the mythical. Some philosophers, including Susan Langer, have argued that these three experiential realms come from the same source: mythic consciousness.

One of my philosophy professors, Dr. Thomas Early, introduced his Philosophy of Aesthetics classes to the writings of Susan Langer, specifically her work entitled, "Feeling and Form."[40] Many times since, I have come to this work and others by her to seek understanding of aesthetic processes and fully-grown experiences only dimly addressed by logical or linear thinking. Specifically, Langer, when exploring the mental origin and function of artistic expression, says:

"Non-discursive[41] form in art has a different office, namely to articulate knowledge that cannot be rendered discursively because it concerns experiences that are not formally amenable to discursive projection. Such experiences are the rhythms of life, organic, emotional and mental (the rhythm of attention is an interesting link among them all), which are not simply periodic, but endlessly complex, and sensitive to every sort of influence. All together they compose a dynamic pattern of feeling."[42]

If so, and if dreams are an example of non-discursive experiences, then the examination of dream content is an interdisciplinary venture that includes poetry and other literary sources, and/or they are an art form unto themselves[43].

Relevant to this last claim, Langer continuously makes the argument, while presenting a strong case from Freudian ideas that relate to non-discursive art forms, that poetry and dreams emanate from the same "mythic consciousness," or have a non-linear "poetic meaning." She says:

"Every product of imagination—be it the intelligently organized work of an artist, or the spontaneous fabrication of a dreamer—comes to the recipient as an experience, a qualitative direct datum."

By implication, I deduce then that *this sort of primal experiencing and expressing of life processes are qualitatively more pure because their origin is more authentic, and in the case of dreams never synthetic, emanating during uncensored affirmations or creative reconstitutions of cognitive and experiential data.* More importantly, because Langer assumes or agrees with others that non-discursive principles of expression equally apply to or govern "the formation of dreams, mythical conceits, and the virtual construction of art," then her thesis echoes an often-recognized bridge between artistic expression and some forms mental instability, a vulnerability that might even extend into our own SP/LD experiences when these are not known (see Chapter Four). She asks the important question, "What, then, really sets poetry apart from dream and neurosis," a question I am now willing to pursue as well.

Correctly so, I think, her question and answer finally distinguishes poetic expression from dreams and neurosis on the basis of "purpose." As she deduces this important distinguishing feature, *purpose*, she writes:

"the poet knows and wishes to set forth by the only symbolic form that will express it. A poem is not, like a dream, a proxy for literal ideas, intended to hide wishes and feelings from oneself and others; it is meant to be always emotionally transparent. Like all deliberate expression, it meets a public standard of excellence. One does not say of a sleeper that he dreams clumsily . . . The process of poetic organization is not a spontaneous association of images, words, situations, and emotions, all amazingly interwoven, without effort, through the unconscious activity Freud called 'the dream work.'"

I think that Susan Langer hits the nail on the head when she singles out "purposeful" behavior as the distinguishing characteristic between art and neurosis[44]. It is unfortunate that neither Langer nor Freud experienced sleep paralysis or lucid dreams, for if they had, they would have agreed that at least some types of dreams are more "purposeful" than others. Interestingly, no lucid dreamers I know, particularly those who pursue LD as a significant and creative activity in their lives, think that the doings of LD are without "purpose" or can be accessed "without effort." In this respect, the purposeful seeking of these states, their manipulation and control, their richer creative possibilities unrestrained by natural laws, are even superior forms of 'poesis'.

I also disagree with Langer that "spontaneity" is not a component of poetic expression, especially when poetry utilizes post-experiential and literal methods to prolong the spontaneity of a certain original feeling or experience. African calling out song and verse exchanges and Haiku poetry are spontaneous compositions, the latter even being connected with a pure moment of enlightenment[45]. I further disagree with Langer that all dreams are simply a "proxy for literal ideas" or always "hide wishes and feelings" and ask in turn: *What if dreaming is composed, deliberate, and can be judged by a public? Doesn't dreaming, particularly that of the SP and LD types, then become a form of poetry itself? Lucid dreaming in this sense, if we are remembering these experiences correctly after waking up, is a form of poetry.*

There is another analysis found in Langer that makes SP/LD experiences if not equal at least similar to poetry. Langer, again using Freudian dream constructs, writes about another non-discursive principle in art expression that Freud referred to as "over-determination" that Langer analyses to mean and include a *principle of ambivalence* where two seemingly opposing thoughts and feelings co-exist and convey an artistic sense. In her examples, poetry as art simultaneously expresses, or can express, exclusionary dichotomies found in logical discourse or the scientific method, such as joy-grief, joy-melancholy, or desire-fear. Equally important, especially with respect to our earlier description of the "stranger" in

Chapter Two as a semiotically ambiguous invitation to the uncanny, Langer explains their intimate relationship when she observes that, "Small shifts of expression can bring them together, and show their intimate relations to each other, whereas literal description can only emphasize their separateness. Where there is no exclusion of opposites, there is also, strictly speaking, no negative. In non-verbal arts this is obvious; omissions may be significant but never as negatives. In literature, the words, "no," "not," "never," etc., occur freely; but what they deny is thereby created. In poetry there is no negation, but only contrast." As Ms. Gillis' narrative will illustrate, and the contributions of many other subjects confirms, the paralysis during an SP event and the flying occurring while in LD can be two aspects or sides of the same continuum and experience. Both are manifested with equal intensity, the paralysis anticipating and making LD flying even more surreal, not as its negation but as a liberating contrast. While in a lucid dream, the dreamer may also recognize that being heavy footed and lethargic is really a prelude to a glide or a hover. The very opportunity of being in control or not is another contrast and theme. Langer ends this analysis with the observation that, "in poetry there is no genuine logical argument; this again is paralleled by the spaciousness of reasoning in dreams." It is this "spaciousness of reasoning in dreams" when coupled with the element of self-awareness and purpose that makes our uncanny dreams a form of poetry.

To sum up our discussion, our thesis could be put into this manifold thesis format. To the extent that the SP and LD experiences:

1) Are embedded in the *mythical* or in the ancestral *ecological unconscious*
2) Predate logical discourse
3) Are both spontaneous *and* planned

4) Can be learned and expanded as skills
5) Gift the dreamer with kaleidoscopic thought and feeling possibilities
6) Are full of ambiguity and contrasting elements then one has to conclude any of these points:

   a) Either LD *dreamers are themselves poems* (instead of a 'dreaming body' we should begin referring to it as a dreaming-poem)
   b) Or the dreamer is the only true poet
   c) Or so-called "pure poetry" can only be achieved while in these or similar states
   d) Or LD is a form of poetry (can be taught, can be learned, etc.)

I would need an entire book to make a full-fledged case for my answer that in fact SP/LD states of dreaming are a type of poetry and as such it would be as strange to approach these as sleep dysfunctions as to treat poets for composing verse. In contrast to the above aesthetic and favorable interpretation of dreaming as poetry, another alternative would be that these experiences might give rise, unintentionally, to mental dysfunction. But even then, doesn't the clinician need to be well versed in the mythical language of the dream world of the patient? The short answer that I have heard from a handful of psychiatrists is: medicate. But the poet, a poet is born, and will soon be doing nightly mischief in the uncanny.

I shall concede one point only tangentially addressed by Langer; namely that LD states usually, not always, don't last very long and in this respect they are more like Haiku poetry than long ancient mariner types of poems. The consolation prize for the short duration of these experiences is how intensely felt these experiences can be, the possibility for increasing their occurrence, and of course, the possibility of control. The fact that the LD experience is limited to REM periods makes learning it as a skill akin to trying to learn how to ride a bicycle during extremely short bursts of time[46]. In many frustrated instances, at least at the onset of learning the skill, the experience is more like mounting and dismounting a bicycle with little time to pedal in between. In other situations, we think we are ready to mount and pedal only to find that someone switched our bicycle and replaced with a unicycle! Regardless, the transitory nature of SP and LD states might even increase our appreciation for them, poetically speaking, in the same manner as a pithy but revealing poem might, or a lovely song fades within minutes, being mesmerized by a rainbow, swallowing a gulp of extraordinary wine, or capturing a fleeting look of a loved one can be all be 'transitory'.

But infinitely much better than philosophical analyses, scientific second-guessing, or my own commentaries about these aesthetic ideas, would be to read a different and authentic voice speaking about SP and LD at length. What follows is a verbatim account by Ms. Gillis. I have opted not to comment on her contribution now by interrupting the flow of her narrative. Rather, I will make use of her observations and examples in subsequent chapters as important points of illustration.

Sleep Paralysis and Lucid Dreaming: A Personal Account, By Lucy Gillis

Sleep was never anything to fear. When I was a child I had very few nightmares, and even those were pretty brief and mild. I didn't pay much attention to dreams then, though I know I could recall them easily. Sometimes, when drifting off to sleep, I'd hear people talking, or see brief images. I'd still feel like I was awake, though very sleepy. I figured that the sounds and images were just the beginnings of dreams, so I didn't pay much attention to them either.

Every now and then I'd get that "jerking awake" sensation, or the sensation of falling, that would wake me suddenly. I'd be startled for a moment, but never frightened by it. Going to sleep was usually effortless and sometimes even fun, in that I'd play with my consciousness. Consciousness is not quite the right word, but I don't know what else to call it. To be honest, I didn't call it by any term at that time. I never talked to anyone about it.

While I would lie in bed, I could create a sensation, at will, of swinging inside and yet not inside my head. It felt like my inner headspace was massive, huge, and totally dark. Of course my eyes would be closed at the time, so that may have accounted for the absence of imagery. I would feel like I was on a huge invisible swing and was swinging back and up, as though towering a great distance above my body, yet I didn't feel separate from my body. I never considered that I could swing out of my body. It never occurred to me. I would swing back and forth in this peaceful dark space over and over until I'd fall asleep. It was fun and somehow relaxing.

As I grew older, this "mind swing" sensation became less frequent, probably because I had more important things on my mind as I was growing up. I continued to recall my dreams, but still didn't pay much attention to them. However, one incident remains in my memory, because it was so different from anything I had experienced before. One day when I was in my late teens, I had fallen asleep on my bed, on top of the bedclothes. I "woke" to find that I couldn't move, and that someone had gotten into the house. I could hear whoever it was coming upstairs toward my bedroom. I could see the open doorway at the foot of my bed and I fully expected to see someone come through it. I was terrified, and tried to scream, but nothing would come out of my mouth, I couldn't even move my mouth. No matter how much I struggled, I couldn't budge. The more I fought to get up or scream, the more intense my fear became. Within moments, however, I was suddenly able to move and I got up quickly, to find with relief that no one had been coming up the stairs at all.

I couldn't recall anything like that ever happening before. I was curious, but not overly frightened by the event. Being unable to move was a bit of a mystery though. Since I wasn't prone to nightmares and wasn't used to them, I assumed it must have been a nightmare of some sort and that I had just been too scared to move. I didn't give it any more thought.

In my mid-twenties I developed an interest in consciousness studies, and became intrigued with dreams and meditative states of consciousness. I remembered my "mind swinging" from childhood. Indeed, I could still do it now and then.

I read about out-of-body experiences, or OBEs, but since I had never had one I was skeptical about what exactly it was that other people were experiencing. Perhaps they were just extremely vivid dreams. It didn't occur to me that my "mind swing" closely matched some descriptions of pre-OBE sensations.

During this time I also learned about lucid dreaming, and it fascinated me to no end to think that you could bring your waking consciousness into the dream state and then be able to direct and manipulate your dreams, if you chose to, while your body slept. You could have just about any adventure you wanted: walk through walls, fly, go into outer space, indulge in fantasies. The list seemed endless. I was very intrigued by all this and hoped that I would one day be able to "go lucid" myself.

I didn't have to wait very long. Within a few months I had my first lucid dream and I was hooked! I wanted more! What a rush to be awake and aware in my dreams, while my body was sleeping!

Eventually I also had what I could only describe as an out-of-body experience and I then knew beyond a doubt that what others were describing were definitely not just vivid dreams. There was a striking difference.

I also discovered that the disjointed images and sounds I

sometimes experienced just on the edge of sleep—that I thought were the "beginnings of dreams"—had a name, hypnagogia, and that it was quite common. Hypnopompia was the same thing, but at the end of sleep, just at the edge of waking. The sleep and dream states were becoming more and more fascinating to me.

As my interest grew, I continued to read as much as I could on the subject of lucid dreams, OBEs, and the sleep cycles that we all go through every night. I learned that during the REM cycle, the body is essentially paralyzed (except for the eyes, which are moving, hence the term Rapid Eye Movement, or REM, to mark this phase). While I was reading and studying the literature about lucid dreams and OBEs I eventually came across the phenomenon of conscious awareness during the sleep paralysis phase. I immediately recalled the episode in my teen years of waking and not being able to move. So that's what that was, I thought to myself. Mystery solved.

During these years I also developed a correspondence with several lucid dreamers and was quite intrigued by their personal dream experiences. One of the women I corresponded with was a very skilled lucid dreamer. We sent each other written descriptions of our lucid dreams on a regular basis. I learned so much from her explorations into the sleep state and dream world.

After a time, she decided it would be fun and informative to begin an exchange of lucid dreams amongst interested dreamers. We sent our written dream reports to her and she put them all together in a booklet format and mailed copies to each of us. Another friend, and equally accomplished lucid dreamer and OBE experiencer, suggested the name "The Lucid Dream Exchange".

The LDE, as we all came to call it, was a valuable source of information for me. So many people were having such wonderful adventures and performing exciting experiments in their lucid dreams. It was a great source of inspiration and encouragement, and was quite educational for me since I was so new to the field.

From reading through the submitted dreams, it was obvious that there were many levels of lucidity—low levels where one is vaguely aware that one is dreaming, to high levels where one knows fully that the entire experience is happening in the dream state and where one recalls waking life with ease and accuracy. Some lucid dreamers seemed to be aware of their dream and their sleeping body at the same time[47].

I was particularly intrigued by this dual sense of awareness. Having conscious awareness in the dream state (lucid dreaming) was fascinating. Having awareness of one's physical body while still asleep and dreaming was even more fascinating to me. My ideas of perception and the senses were changing.

Within time, I experienced this dual awareness for myself and was delighted that I could be in a dream, aware that I was dreaming in a dream body, and yet still feel sensations in my physical body. I felt thrilled to have my consciousness in such a delicate yet powerful balance between waking and dreaming realities. This happened again on several occasions, the following simple scene being one of the most vivid:

"I practically had to hurl myself out of bed, it was so hard to move. I staggered quickly out to the hall, wondering if I was really awake. Perhaps I was still dreaming. While standing in the hallway, I wiggled my hip and was surprised to feel the body pillow against my real hip in the bed. Amazingly, I was standing in the dimly lit hallway feeling my dream hip wiggle while I was simultaneously in the cozy bed, feeling the body pillow against my hip."

This kind of dual awareness seemed to be similar to what some people were experiencing in the sleep paralysis state: they were dreaming, aware of their dream imagery, yet they were also feeling sensations that seemed to be in their physical sleeping bodies.

From the contributors to LDE, and in other literature, I also read accounts of what is now usually referred to as "classic" out-of-body sensations and awareness during sleep paralysis. The classic OBE and sleep paralysis sensations included such things as loud buzzing or roaring noises; vibrations or energy running through the body; a heaviness on the chest; difficulty breathing; inability to move; sometimes even the feeling of a presence in the room; auditory and/or visual hallucinations; and usually a high degree of terror, particularly if the dreamer didn't know what was really happening. In many of the sources I read, these symptoms were often depicted as an incubus or demon sitting on the dreamer's chest.

Some descriptions, namely of the visual and auditory hallucinations, resembled the disjointed dream fragments of hypnagogia and hypnopompia. Most of these reports stated that these "symptoms" were occurring either at the beginning of sleep or more commonly, at the end, near the point of waking. One of my favorite definitions of sleep paralysis is that your mind wakes up just before your body does.

I am lucky in that whenever I read or hear about something related to consciousness or dreaming that I haven't experienced before, my curiosity and desire to experience it for myself is strong enough to induce the event. Or perhaps desire has nothing to do with it at all. Maybe because I am suddenly aware of something new, I am then able to imagine it, and hence able to do it.

By now I had experienced several out-of-bodies, but I had never felt those "classic" sensations prior to having an OBE. Outside of my teenage experience of waking and not being able to move, I hadn't experienced awareness of sleep paralysis either. I was kind of jealous. I wanted to know what these classic symptoms felt like. Eventually, I began to experience some of them—surely due to my intense curiosity, the power of suggestion, and my ever-present desire to know more about sleep and dreaming.

———

However, my curiosity was swiftly satisfied and my jealously vanished when I realized that it could still be somewhat frightening even when you knew what was really happening:

"As I try to sleep I feel a weird sensation, as though my whole body is turning to stone. It is especially noticeable on my face. I feel the muscles tighten, my lip twitches and I feel a pulling sensation, as though someone is pulling my upper lip to the left. It also feels like there is a thickening—like a thigh forming—between my legs. Probably the pillow, I think to myself (I usually sleep with a pillow between my knees). I begin to get nervous even though I know this must be sleep paralysis coming on. I struggle to wake up. I open my eyes (dream eyes?) very slightly. I can't open them all the way. It's so hard to move. I know I should just relax into it and so I take a deep breath and try to do so. Soon though, I am struggling again. Once more I try relaxing and it feels much better. During this time I hear a rushing, like wind, passing all around my body but I don't feel the sensation of wind on my body. This lasts for quite a while. I finally pull myself out of it and go into a false awakening (a dream in which you believe you have awakened, but in fact you haven't). At one point I hear a loud buzzing/crackling noise, which seems to be outside my bedroom window. I have no idea what it is and I am too nervous to get up and look out."

After this incident, I decided that I didn't really need to experience the so-called classic symptoms in order to become lucid or to have an OBE, or to be like other people. I realized that I was lucky that I could have lucid dreams and the occasional OBE fairly easily without anxiety or fear. Besides, dwelling on it, expecting it, and desiring to experience these things only seemed to draw them to me. Since I didn't need classic OBE symptoms before, why bring them on purposely now? So I dropped my desire to experience them. They didn't disappear altogether, but their occurrences were rare.

As the years went on and I had more experiences with lucid dreaming and OBEs my rather rare episodes of sleep paralysis sensations could still provoke a little anxiety, but were more often than not quite interesting to experience.

Since I knew what was occurring, I would try to remain calm. By being calm and allowing the experience to unfold or pass, as it were, the sleep paralysis effects were over quickly and I felt no more fear or anxiety. Sometimes, however, I'd struggle, out of habit or reflex. Even though I knew it was only "dream stuff" the adrenaline was already pumping.

I later discovered in reading accounts in LDE and through my own experience that awareness of sleep paralysis was not limited to the onset or ending of sleep. Sometimes it could be experienced in the middle of a lengthy dream. I found there were many lucid dreamers who seemed to sense the effects of sleep paralysis during their lucid dreams, as they briefly identified with their sleeping bodies. This would often manifest as difficulty moving or breathing in their dream. Instead of getting caught up in the dream drama, most dreamers would simply acknowledge the sensations, chalk them up to sleep paralysis, and either ignore them or wait for them to pass.

Some dreamers even manipulated the sensations, and due to reading about other dreamers' playfulness, my curiosity was piqued and I wanted to try it too:

"It is night time and I'm walking along narrow, empty streets. I am almost lucid in that I know that I'm creating the scene around me, and yet I wonder when I will see a building or storefront that I recognize. The streets are very hilly and I feel I have been walking for quite a while. Then my awareness shifts to my body on the bed. I don't know if I woke or if it was a false awakening, but I assumed the previous image of walking down the streets was hypnagogic imagery or a disjointed dream fragment.

The next thing I know, I feel a cold wind across my curled up legs. I open my eyes (or were they my dream eyes?) and see my right pajama-

*clad thigh exposed, not under the bed covers. I'm on my left side. I am
so sleepy, I let my eyes close. But I recognize the wind as a pre-OBE—
sleep paralysis phenomenon. I will the wind to get stronger and colder.
It also gets louder as I hear it roaring past my curled up body. I even
wonder if it will strip my leg naked, it seems so rough and harsh. I
wonder if the "feeling" of the cold wind will somehow translate as a
symbol of "nakedness." I can't seem to think of the word "dream"
although I know what it means. I don't struggle to remember the word,
I think it will wake me if I try too hard.*

*Suddenly I remind myself, Hey I'm doing this! Why am I
concentrating on a cold wind? I want a warm wind! A tropical
breeze! I briefly think of palm trees, blue skies, and a white sandy
beach, in an effort to change the wind. The wind dies down and warms
up a little, but it is still a cold wind. I try to move, but I can't budge.
Now I'm certain I am in sleep paralysis. I wait for a few moments,
and then slowly I am able to move a little, then a little more. I wiggle
my arms and legs, struggling a bit to get out of the bed. I momentarily
think I have really awakened and it is my real body that I am moving,
but I soon realize that I'm still dreaming . . ."*

I realized that I could use the sleep paralysis state to help
me recognize when I was dreaming, and that I could remain in
the dream state and not have to wake up. Other dreamers were
writing about this too—how they would then take advantage of
the situation to launch themselves into lucid dreams or OBEs.
One of my most intriguing experiences with sleep paralysis
during a dream occurred one evening when I took a brief nap:

*"I am sitting on a bed in my childhood bedroom. It is nighttime.
I get up and look out the west-facing window, craning my neck to be
able to see my grandmother's place up on the hill. It is all in darkness
up there. I know it must be around 6:00 p.m. and I guess that they
are in the living room watching the news and haven't turned on the
kitchen lights yet. I look up into the sky at the brilliant stars.*

Then it seems I am laying in the bed again. I get up, feeling groggy, and find it difficult to open my eyes. I touch my face and am startled to find it is swollen. My head feels numb. I put my hands to my head and discover that my whole head is swollen. I feel my swollen face, and my glasses, and I get a bit panicked, wondering briefly how I am able to breathe. I stumble into the hall trying to call for D in the next room, knowing he will get me to a hospital where I can get some help. I can't talk. My ears tingle, and I still can't open my eyes fully. I can just barely make out light paneled walls in the wide hallway when my eyes crack open for a split second.

Then I slow down, and decide I must still be asleep and these sensations are the result of sleep paralysis. I know that relaxing will reduce the sensations, and possibly eliminate them. Soon I get the sensation of laying in bed and I think to myself that this would be a good time to try for a lucid dream or out-of-body. But I am so tired, I don't really feel like exerting any effort. However, in the next instant, I feel as though I am a black/dark purple, thick liquid/mist in the outline of a human body. (I feel I am in this body and yet I am observing it as though laying beside it.) I sit up, thinking about sitting up and leaving my physical body laying down. It feels like I have done this.

Then suddenly I hear the theme music and see a brief scene from the opening of an old TV show from the 70's "Love, American Style." Just as quickly as the music and scene appear, it is gone and I begin to slowly rotate upwards (as though doing a backward somersault in the air), my (liquid/mist) legs in the air first. With my legs still higher than the rest of me, I twist, like a corkscrew, into my physical body, feeling then like a small dry mist, or smoke (light purple or mauve) curling inside the head and upper portion of my body, as I settle/dissolve into my physical body. (I don't maneuver like this intentionally, it is all very automatic.) I wake, stretch, and ensure that I am able to talk and move my jaw, my head feeling normal and not swollen at all. I am delighted to have had such a strange and intriguing experience."

It is encouraging to know that some sleep paralysis feelings experienced in the dream state can go from strange and frightening to intriguing and fun, once you know what is happening, and that you can't be hurt. It can be a great gateway to lucid dreaming or out-of-body adventures.

Many lucid dreamers, (myself included) notice that their thoughts and expectations affect the content of their dreams.

While studying lucid dreaming and altered states of consciousness I was coming to believe strongly in the philosophy that "You Create Your Own Reality." In other words you create your own experience of personal reality by your beliefs, expectations, attitudes, and emotions. I found this easy to believe in the light of dream experiences. My dreams followed faithfully my expectations and beliefs, however subtly they may have appeared at first.

I feel that this belief has helped me to keep my rare experiences of sleep paralysis from becoming too nightmarish. Indeed, I'm sure this firm belief has also helped me to keep any kind of nightmare from fully developing. Besides, now that I know what sleep paralysis is, this knowledge alone renders the situation be less frightening than it otherwise could be.

In some lucid dreams, if I would find myself beginning to feel fearful (maybe after watching a scary movie before sleeping), I would remind myself that my fears and emotions could create fearful dream imagery and therefore, if I came across anything frightening in the dream, I should remember that it was a reflection, a symbol of my own fears. As I expected, my dreams co-operated beautifully and on one occasion presented a humorous symbol to show me that indeed, my expectations were creating my dream experience:

"I walk down the hallway and I wonder if I am dreaming. I try to fly. I feel a ripple through my body that I call a "dream chill" as my attempt to fly succeeds. I fly a bit, then penetrate the kitchen

window. I glide over the grass smoothly, my belly just touching. It is a windy, sunny day. I have trouble flying in the wind (no doubt because I expected to).

Soon I am in sitting in a building. I still know I'm dreaming. I feel kind of nervous. I get up and stomp my feet as I walk, and slap my hands together loudly as I sing, hoping the noise and movement will shake off my nervous feelings. It feels like I've been "brought" here somehow. I discover that I'm naked. The place is full of offices, but is empty of people. I'm all alone.

I go into one area around a corner. Three of the "walls" are either made of curtains or have curtains over them. There is a desk with a lit lamp on it to my left. I lay on the desk. Looking up at the lamp makes me think of an alien examination room, where big-eyed aliens would peer down on me, and I get up quickly and say something like "You're trying to make me feel comfortable here," (by making the place resemble ordinary offices) to any "alien" that may be listening.

I walk and sing and clap my hands even louder than before. I'm feeling a bit more uneasy, I wonder if my fear will create scary alien imagery. I try to drop that idea. Then suddenly I see a man strolling nonchalantly by. He "looks" like K from work and I say "Hi K!" I am a little surprised to see that he has no face, just skin where his features should be. He has hair and wears a hat, but has no face. I know this is because of my recent thought—that I didn't want to create a scary big-eyed alien. I am pleased and amused that my mind produced a harmless, faceless image, in response to my attempts to let go of fearful feelings and thoughts."

This served to strengthen my belief that my dream experiences were largely influenced by my thoughts. So to manifest positive imagery and scenarios, remaining calm and turning my attention away from negative or frightening thinking was the secret. At least for me.

I had many other dreams like the one above in which by simply recognizing that my thoughts and expectations could create distressing situations, I discovered time and again, that by making the effort to change or let go of fearful thoughts dramatically reduced their chances of causing fearful dream imagery.

I was aware that this really wasn't a new idea. In the lucid dreaming literature I had found many references to the fact that some therapists and psychologists were using lucid dreaming as part of their prescribed therapy for nightmare sufferers. If the patients could learn to recognise that they were dreaming, they could then make some choices as to how to handle the nightmare. Reports seemed to indicate that there was a lot of success in this area, particularly with children.

Eventually I became co-editor and publisher of The Lucid Dream Exchange, and have since read hundreds of lucid dream and OBE reports from people of all walks of life. I am constantly amazed by the depth and variety of experiences that dreamers have. Their sense of adventure and drive for exploration are a real inspiration.

I've noticed that most of the sleep paralysis reports that readers have submitted to LDE don't seem to be of the terrifying variety. Some of the classical symptoms are there, but the level of fear or anxiety is fairly low. I believe there may be several reasons for this. Certainly, since the tone of the LDE is a positive one, perhaps readers are reluctant to send in nightmarish dream reports. Another factor may be that since these readers are interested in lucid dreaming they are probably more educated in the stages of the sleep cycle than the average person; therefore, they are able to recognize sleep paralysis when it occurs. Many also realize that their thoughts and beliefs largely influence their dreams and when lucid they make the effort to be more positive and calm. Also, because of their desire for lucidity in dreams, they welcome awareness during sleep and take advantage of it when it occurs, instead of struggling to wake up.

An avid interest in lucid dreaming, namely the desire to bring waking consciousness into the dream state, offers a great opportunity to experience awareness of other phases of the sleep cycle, in particular the sleep paralysis stage.

I believe that those who experience sleep paralysis are a step ahead of those who do not and who want to experience lucid dreaming or out-of-body explorations. The sleep paralysis "sufferer" is experiencing what the lucid dreamer strives for: awareness during sleep.

I would encourage those who occasionally experience awareness during sleep paralysis to first learn to overcome or at least minimize their fear response to their situation. Once this has been achieved, I would recommend that dreamers then try to carry their awareness into the dream state.

Once lucid, the adventures a dreamer can have are limited only by the dreamer's imagination—flights of fancy, walking on water, flying, acting out fantasies, whatever the dreamer desires. I hope that everyone who is prone to awareness during sleep paralysis will learn to initiate lucid dreaming, to step away from the fear and terror and move beyond to wonderful and exciting dream adventures.

Sleep should never be anything to fear.

Out of Phase Dual Awareness? By Lucy Gillis

I had an idea occur to me when I read of a sleep paralysis incident experienced by Jorge Conesa. During an e-mail discussion, Jorge wrote:

"I induced an SP and accidentally an OBE three nights ago. I panicked seeing my own body and did not know how to get back. So I approached my sleeping body and began chewing on and biting my own toes so I would wake up. This did not work. So instead, I did my "roll up" trick[48] and woke up with a jolt!

It struck me funny and I burst out laughing at the thought of being OBE, hunched over your own physical body and gnawing on your own feet! A comical image indeed! But then, that image of a hunched figure bent over a sleeping body led me to recall some of the classical nightmare descriptions, such as an incubus crouched on a sleeper's chest, the familiar image often used when describing effects of sleep paralysis.

And then I began to wonder... What if, on some occasions, the dreamer himself is the one actively producing the sensations felt during sleep paralysis?

Suppose the dreamer doesn't recall being out of body. According to one theory, we leave our bodies every night when we sleep. We simply don't remember that we do so. Just like we all dream every night, but not everyone remembers their dreams. (For those who don't believe that we "go" anywhere in our sleep, instead of the phrase "leave our bodies," substitute "withdraw attention from the outer physical environment as our senses become cut off or reduced as we enter the sleep cycle.")

Add to this the fact that time does not usually operate in the dream state as it does in waking reality. In some dreams, hours or days can be felt to pass when in fact only moments have gone by. What if, besides this time distortion, there can sometimes also be a time lag? What if our bodies experience sensations that may have had their origin only seconds *before*, but the cause of those sensations (the dream) is forgotten, like some out-of-phase dual awareness?

Could this be a kind of dual awareness, but not a strictly simultaneous one? Could sensations being produced during the dream scene be felt physically *after* the scene is over?

Feelings and emotions are often more easily recalled when we awaken than are visual images. I'm sure we've all on occasion awakened from a dream with a lingering feeling, perhaps anxiety, or happiness, yet we couldn't recall what the specific dream was about.

What if, in the out of body state, we encounter difficulties getting back into the physical body? (Or, if not "out of body" we encounter difficulties in waking up and we hallucinate a dream version of our waking body.) What if we do like Jorge and attempt to get back in (or wake up) by alerting the physical body, trying to stir it to wakefulness? Could some of the sensations felt during sleep paralysis be an "echo" of this activity when the mind switches from dreaming consciousness to waking?

If we tend not to remember our dreams when we wake, or not recall out of body excursions, but we have a lasting feeling of anxiety or panic (from trying to get back in the body or wake up), perhaps the mind produces a distorted version of what is happening, trying to translate the sensations into something familiar, as best it can.

Could we ourselves be the "demon" sitting on our own chests, trying to get back into our bodies, when in fact it is the mind trying to translate the dream experience of our own attempts to return to waking reality?[49]

"A Dynamic Pattern of Feeling": A Lucid Dream, By Jorge Conesa

In 1993 I was trying to decide if I could afford to pursue post-graduate work or whether it was better to become employed to start paying my student loans. A position to teach in the Pacific Northwest opened up and necessity won out; I took the job. In retrospect, this was an excellent opportunity and I have benefited immensely from taking this path. As it turns out, that decision has directly impacted the writing of this book in that the increased freedom found in a smaller academic setting, without the strings-attached and publish-or-perish academic mode and frenzy of alternative routes, has given me more quality time to *do the uncanny*, and to think about and devote my interests to the SP/LD phenomenon. While in the midst of this decision-making I had three lucid dreams on three consecutive nights (the dreams were vivid, in color, with sounds).

First Night

I am walking on snow, and I hear the snow crushing under my weight and footsteps. I realize that I am dreaming, that this is a lucid dream, so I start paying close attention to everything happening around me. I keep walking on the snow in a birch forest until I come to a shelter made of animal skins. The shelter is about 12 feet wide by 30 feet long and possibly as high as 7-8 feet. The shelter is shaped as a half cylinder with tapering and protruding ends. It is animal like. I stop at the entrance to this lodge; I pull the skin-door open and then I wake up. I feel the hairs left on the skin and these feel soft to the touch.

Second Night

I start lucid dreaming in the same place I started the previous night. But now, I have a goal: I am curious about what's inside the lodge. So I walk again on the snow hearing the crushing sound under my feet (which, by the way, are covered with skin leggings—something I did not observe the pervious night) until I reach the lodge. I grab the skin-flap and door, pull it aside (right-to-left) and enter the lodge. It is very dark inside but I can see that there are a couple of small fires burning. They look like the yellow fiery eyes of a wolf. I am immediately aware that there are several individuals sitting against the sides of the lodge as if they are waiting for me. As my eyes get used to the darkness, I notice that there are six elderly men on either side of the central walkway, and that there is another elder at the very end of this central walkway. I concentrate on their faces. They look ancient, dark-skinned (possibly Native American, but could be European too, Simi). They are all wearing variations of fur garments of different animals. Some wear fur caps, some don't. I don't feel threatened at all by them; because it really seems to me that they have been waiting for me, that they are there to help me. Although their body language and general demeanor is neutral, I sense that they have good wishes toward me. I keep walking to the end of the lodge until I am facing the 13th elder at the back of the lodge. He is also very old. He looks at me and pulls out a leather pouch. I wake up.

Third Night

The exact chain of events from the previous night is repeated. The unfolding of these events seems to take the same time as it took the two previous nights. But on this night, the 13th elder pulls out three objects from his leather pouch: a lapis lazuli shiny sphere, a pyrite pyramid, and a cube made out of marble or alabaster. He grabs my hand (I don't remember which) and deposits all three objects there. I have to spread wide and extend all my fingers to hold onto these objects because they are not small. I look at the three objects for a long time reminding myself to pay close attention to detail and try to extend my concentration as long as I can. Finally, I wake up.

Interpretation of "A Dynamic Pattern of Feeling"

I decided to pursue teaching shortly after this last dream. A few months later my wife, a Montessori educator, started getting the journal, *Montessori Life*, and I was surprised to see that their logo is a triangle, a square, and a circle. (Equally possible, and suggested by my wife who is more skeptical than I, she believes that I had already seen these symbols somewhere in a letterhead. I think that this is equally possible although I was not consciously aware of this at the time.) The meaning derived from this three-part LD could have been very straightforward the, and I might have taken the three shapes to symbolize teaching. However, perhaps more convoluted interpretations are possible.

As the years pass and I revisit this uncanny experience additional information trickles in and make that memory richer. For example, I have learned since then that in Montessori education the three basic shapes and their exact sequence in the AMS logo (triangle, circle, and square) are first introduced early in preschool as a sensorial material. Montessori children learn to trace the shapes of these polygons with their fingers and, in order to achieve maximum tactile contrast, they first trace the triangle then move to the circle and move again to another dramatic contrast gradient by touching the square. Going back to Freud's *Principle of Ambivalence*, these shape differences are not in opposition to each other but represent a fundamental contrast: all polygons derive from the circle-polygon so they are contained within it even though they may look like different shapes. Additional relationships that hold together in meaning, in a complex numerical semiotic web, are the facts that: i) the first three digits of the number Pi (3.14) are numerical representations of the triangle, the circle (the last polygon or the "whole," the one), and the square, and Pi appears in the exact Montessorian sequence; ii) of course, Jesus and the twelve disciples is an example of the universal motif and council of thirteen elders—the twelve elders and a thirteenth elder-leader make a traditional council and suggest an ongoing democratic process that in both represent a teaching forum as well; and iii) multiplying *three* times *four* and adding *one* (the thirteenth elder) equals thirteen. These elements taken ensemble represent basic knowledge, or the way knowledge is thought about and transmitted, and overall, an obvious direction toward continued learning and teaching.

Additional interpretations include both overt and covert elements; for example, the conjuring of a winter dreamscape coincided perhaps with the coming of winter in Ohio. But also, in Langer's observation of contrast and ambivalence in poetry, the snow-covered landscape and the cozy interior of the hut are contrasting a singular fact of human existence and their appreciation or rejection can only occur by having both perspectives. In the LD both were equally comforting. The Native American atmosphere element, and more importantly, seeing it as ultimate wisdom, is something dear to my childhood—my admiration of authentic, natural and ancient ways. But this element was also archetypical or generic in that no particular ethnic group was prominent. Another generic, even universal motif was that of "secrets hidden in pouches" and their contents as stones, minerals, botanical or even animal parts. The three objects and their shapes have also been used universally or locally to convey perceived universal truths. Spheres and circles can stand for symbols of the Self, according to Jung, or to journeys to be started or to be completed or to signify an eternal cycle. The womb is the first sphere associated with birth and with a beginning. Cubes and squares (four-sided or eight-sided motifs) have been employed to signify four or more directions, each offering a different perspective, mood or 'wind'. Pyramids and triangles equally convey stability, strength, directionality, and cycles.

The act of receiving rather than rejecting these shapes as they are placed in my hand indicate a plethora of truths about myself: accepting a final and authoritative prescription if the source is genuine; assuming that somehow I was part of the choice because I chose to go on and receive the judgment; I am ready to move on and start on a new journey; the very idea of authoritative "truth" as being enigmatic in the end, or at least open-ended; the fact that truth can be found if one is really looking for "it" and willing to accept what it has to offer; and last but not least, the final vault that might enclose "truth" not being a vault at all but something as flimsy, malleable and shifting as a leather pouch, too fragile to contain important ideas.

Any of these symbols alone is ambiguous enough, and together they either produce added ambiguity or give rise to a specific message whose syntax I was able to discern or interpret at my own convenience or benefit. And always, any of these motifs are part of my ontological development at unconscious and conscious levels. Is this poetry? It felt more like art cinema, but yes, it can be. The dream-as-a-poem, translated now into the imperfect realm of words-as-a-poem, may have sounded something like this:

A white-tall, white-below, white-around forest calls
And draws the seeker into a clearing.
The house-wolf, long and lanky,
Stalks with knowledge.
He opens its mouth and feels the warm breath.
Inside the animal are fires and others, thirteen to be exact,
*   with eyes as fires.*
He walks the length of the bowels led by wrinkled-roads,
And ageless faces: a murder of sorcerers.
He now stands at the end, where the fangs don't bite,
And the oldest hand, inserted in a skunk stomach,
Retrieves and forces as an answer:
A blue ball as big as buckwheat;
A fool's gold pyramid, small enough to bury a mantis
*   queen;*
And a marble cube, big enough to damage a skull.
Outside, standing in the real snow, the seeker does the math:
One wolf-tent;
Thirteen breaths;
One Triangle;
A Circle;
One square.
And the answer seems clear.

Epilogue to This Chapter

I have logged a number of these lucid dreams and experiences but this one stands out for some reason more than the others, partly because it came to be seen as an example of dreaming during a specific problem-solving situation and decision that changed the course of our family in a significant way. The three-part lucid dream might have been a catalyst for making a professional decision. The very fact that I had control over these dream sequences probably gave me a sense of control during my waking life, thus allowing me to make a decision, any decision.

It is also a real example of an encounter with the uncanny, with the worlds we enter and the ghosts we wrestle and play with each night. Multiply these dreams and images by millions of dreamers, and their SP/LD dreams and mythology and art become staples of human experience. At the end of this chapter, even when we might be uncomfortable still in referring to dreams as poems we might accept and use Langer's more academic and safer construct for LDs as 'dynamic patterns of feeling.'

Ino Moxo's multidimensional jungle, external and internal, presents limitless opportunities for reflection, acceptance, transformation, and creation. The anthropologist Lévi-Strauss, I believe, would define this set of possibilities as *bricolage*, as a collection of potential signs ready to adopt a useful form whenever needed by the mythical thinker, and in our case, dreamer. Some readers may not ever experience the intensity of these dreamscapes as described above but those of us who do must go on dreaming-living and interpreting. To me, it is far better to view these doings as poetry than as an aberration of sleep, or a sign of dysfunction, or a mere scientific curiosity: these doings can also be all of these, or none. We are faced with an ever present caveat: when we interpret poetry wrongly and believe it, and think that the aliens are real and coming to take away our precious DNA, then it is no longer a case of poetry but of a perverse pamphlet and misguided propaganda. That is the limitation of *bricolage* in that this adaptation and handy collection of signs produces no objective concepts thus there is no way of testing, outside the box, their true reality, if one is immersed in the dream!

I will explore a bit more the value of Lévi-Strauss' concept of *bricolage* for our story in the conclusion. But now, and more relevant to this chapter, I would like to focus on his initial description of this word and application in his French language as: *"a ball rebounding, a dog straying, or a horse swerving from its direct course to avoid an obstacle."* All these behaviors and connotations of the word are descriptions of an inner reality that deviates from an established norm, and manner of thinking that, more and more in this day and age, demands objectivity, palpable facts, and linear thinking in order to establish "truth."

The SP/LD dreamer himself/herself is a *deviant* of this rational and linear thinking trend to the extent that he/she is catapulted into mythical dreaming. Of no fault of his/her own he/she travels back and forth between two audiences and manners of thinking. Like *"a horse swerving to avoid an obstacle,"* as Lévi-Strauss defines *bricolage*, the uncanny dreamer must avoid both the reactions of an intolerant society as well as his/her own inner obstacles. This is what I call a *shamanic journey or task* in the next chapter, and succeeding in this enterprise offers the reward of *becoming* in accelerated way, what Gordon Allport (1955) defines as *saltatory becoming*. In his own words, Allport defines *saltatory becoming* as:

"It sometimes happens that the very center of organization of a personality shifts suddenly and apparently without warning. Some impetus, coming perhaps from a bereavement, an illness, or a religious conversion, even from a teacher or a book, may lead to a reorientation. In such cases of traumatic reentering it is undoubtedly true that the person has latent within him all of the capacities and sentiments that suddenly rise from a subordinate to superordinate position in his being."

Even when the society that the dreamer belongs to openly embraces a mythical realm, it may not be accepting of challenges to traditional interpretations. Such is the case of the mythical orthodoxy of the Zuni, for example, who embrace the opportunity of visionary communion and dream reality as long as it conforms to a strict and *untreatable tradition* of stories and rituals. Such is the case while in the midst of any orthodoxy. As the next chapter charts and Allport described earlier, the potential for psychological instability is great no matter what culture one is in because the reality of uncanny dreaming is first and foremost a subjective reality. There is always, at least an internal struggle with new information, with creating consistency between dreaming and wakeful realms, and with maintaining the integrity of social bonds when the uncanny dreamer speaks of such worlds! Perhaps because this duality of existence, going back to Langer's *principle of ambivalence* or to Freud's *over-determination* where two seemingly opposing thoughts and feelings co-exist, an emerging artistic sense is sometimes the consolation price to this existential predicament. *Poesis* is the reward, the only one I seek at least.

To conclude, the SP/LD experiences may be the closest this agnostic and new shaman explorer will ever get to "cheating death" and to transcend his human form and its physical limitations. If I am in spiritual denial, as some new age friends of mine have characterized my reluctance to facile or trite spirituality, then for me at least, the SP/LD may be my last hope according to them: the cosmos banging on my stupid body and mind letting me in on its secrets. If that is the case, I am fortunate then that my spiritual stupidity has led to so much artistic excitement so soon!

CHAPTER FOUR

A "Shamanic" Map and Territory

"Dreams, from a shamanic point of view, are of two types: ordinary dreams; and nonordinary, or "big" dreams. Shamans are normally only concerned with big dreams. A big dream is a dream that is repeated several times in the same basic way on different nights, or it is a one-time dream that is so vivid that it is like being awake, an unusually powerful dream."

Michael Harner, *The Way of The Shaman*.

The Scientist Shaman

When it comes to the "big" dream of SP, scientist or not, we are all forced into a sort of personal sorcery. It is 'sorcery' from the point of view of the dream content itself (refer to my LD experience and other accounts in this book and in Appendix) to the extent that new frameworks of knowledge exchange are possible beyond the non-dreaming reality. This is simply a fact that must be accepted, and it occurs for millions of individuals on a nightly basis. It is a fact whether my spouse believes it or not; it is fact whether my neighbor believes it or not; it is a fact whether psychological or dream research and science address these experiences adequately or not. Our uncanny "Big" dreams go on manifesting themselves in our psychological reality despite the limitations of dreaming "Big" Dreams elsewhere.

Because these dreams are a unique psychological reality, as well as a significant element of the whole of consciousness and even perhaps the very seeds of what is called the mythical, and because the new frameworks I have suggested employ mythical symbols or occur around ancient themes under the highly impressionable state of the SP/LD experiencer, they gain a certain irrevocability and validity beyond objective science. One can dismiss these knowledge frameworks if one chooses as nothing more than a creative but bizarre state of consciousness,[50] although *noesis* remains. However, this flies in the face of contemporary research on dreaming and REM states that specifically argue for the role of these processes in memory consolidation[51], maintaining a modicum of higher order reasoning states—a pilot light for consciousness if you will—and for problem solving. So at least some of the research shows that cognition is doing something constructive when the lights seem to be out. Generally speaking, though, *it seems that a profound experiential and experimental chasm exists to the extent that the "shaman" specializes in the "Big" dream and most dream research has been devoted instead to the "Little Dream."* This chasm has been almost convenient for both parties, but it does little to bring the entire study of dreams into a singular and ecologically satisfying umbrella. Another falsity, originating in western scientific paradigms of sleep research, is that of dichotomizing consciousness into ordinary versus non-ordinary, or consciousness and altered states of consciousness. I will address this latter limitation at the end of this chapter.

But even when this unfortunate classification, little dreams-big dreams, is addressed in the scientific literature and dream research community, there seems to be little interest, and/or limited personal experience of "Big" dreams. They are just another category of interesting dreams, no more no less. But, even when investigated, "Big" dreams are only inadequately explained, or none at all, by dream theories such as Hobson and McCarley's Activation Synthesis Theory (1977) which views dream events as the result of random activation of medullar and pontine cells. Even when these authors make allowances[52] for the creative abilities of cortical systems to organize this random activation according to some personal agenda and interest, their explanation remains a description of actual dream physiology and only that, since it does not attempt, ecologically speaking, to explain the psychological and cultural regularities of "Big" dreams.

In other words, what others and I call a "mythical" dream language that makes sense to the dreamer, or to a collective of avid vivid dreamers, may be gibberish or the product of random activation to others who, interestingly enough, do not experience SP and LD states and do not understand these experiences no matter how many neuron clusters they investigate. I grudgingly accept and understand their limited position for reasons given in previous chapters, namely, that an experiential chasm exists between the journeyer and the outside, passive, and so-called "objective" observer.

We can put this argument a bit more strongly. In fact, contrary to the orthodoxy of "squeaky clean" dream research, and as an argument against present hyper-technology driven empirical trends in sleep research, I claim that there can be no "objective" or "outside" observer in SP/LD research who does not have an intimate and credible hold on these phenomena. So-called "objective research" can at best be an outside and clouded window into a real and extended phenomenon that can only be understood from an existential and ecologically grander point of view. This is in fact no different than attempting to understand the psychology of "Big" love by studying neuronal activity, hormonal changes, or moist secretions. One has not "captured human love" in an experientially valid sense. Also, there is a phenomenological advantage to the study of love that the study of SP/LD does not have in that we can assume that many more researchers experience love, romantic or otherwise, and can approach their study with a modicum of face validity.

Additionally, to be sure, there is non-randomness in being frozen routinely, or in learning specific rituals/behaviors to induce LD, or even in participating in the exact dream as many times as one wishes. A three-part shamanic lucid dream is anything but random. At the very least, *what these experiences suggest is that, with practice, some less interesting neuronal random activation can be yielded and controlled, once in a state of self-awareness, to enlist the activation of specific brain systems needed to elaborate upon a "Big" dream experience.* If some individuals are capable of doing this, then some of the dream research has to explain how this is accomplished.

To be sure, achieving conscious lucidity or self-awareness sometime during sleep is no small task, but it is theoretically achievable at least if we look at the SP/LD as special cases of extreme consciousness states (See Figure 2) along a continuum begun in no-dreams, passivity, and true randomness dream states. Now, when the SP experiencer is able to produce or manage the circumstances required to achieve a singular event, then he/she possesses, no, owns the non-random story. REM dreaming itself does not "spontaneously" appear "sometime" during the night. Most mammals dream roughly within a 90-minute non-REM—REM cycle; so in this sense, there is nothing random about the "spontaneous" excitement of pontine, and later, sub cortical and cortical areas. What I mean is that this adaptation has a mammalian **purpose** that culminates by a force of **will**, in humans at least, in a singular and repeatable experience: the uncanny dream.

To reiterate, even if we can call these neuronal events "random physiological events" the subsequent cascading effects of this spontaneous cause are further restricted by mental habits and impressions peculiar to the individual and the species. This experiential funnel reduces the scope of randomness even more. Finally, probability is obligated one step beyond when the dreamer dreams "Big Dreams" as a matter of course.

I suppose and can only concede that several acts of "neuronal randomness"[53] end up being a purposeful and singularized non-random event. But the volitional and self-aware quality of SP/LD experiences quickly nullifies an initial and less consequential sort of randomness and makes this psychobiological explanation recede as not very useful for the "shaman" dreamer. LaBerge's (1985) well-known criticisms of Activation Synthesis are reflected in statements like this:

> *"As for meaning and nonsense, the Activation Synthesis model of dreaming seems to completely disregard the possibility . . . that dreams could have any intrinsic or even interesting meaning whatsoever."*

We must agree with his criticism here as well as a major obstacle to any bottom-up theory of dreams which disregards the complexity of a self-aware mind to get to work, for a reason, on any stimulation that goes on during its watch, day or night, or more importantly, a mind that seems to carry intentionality, **purpose**, and goals into the mythic realm of dreaming.

These modern non-experiencing dream-researchers-as-shamans are on to something, but it is a preliminary something at best that may have little or no relevance to the psychological and mythical realms experienced by expert lucid dreamers of all ages. The SP/LD sufferer may regard a clinician and psychologist suspiciously if he/she were to sum up Activation Synthesis as a foundational explanation of how it is that they can engage in conversations with dream entities who provide better counsel.

Is this a failure of reductionism? Is this a confusion about different levels of information processing—one biological, the others experiential-cognitive, psychological or cultural? Is this a failure of embracing cognitvism as an *Information Processing Only* limited paradigm that disregards *meaning processing* and *semiosis*? I think that the level of "information processing" occurring while in these creative states are cognitive for sure, but more importantly, they are also psychological and holistic and cultural, and the pragmatics for managing or expanding these states will not be found in neuron songs, but in the skills of a "sorcerer" or "shaman" dealing with a brand new and uncanny situation, always in a cultural context leading to a number of psychological outcomes. While preserving most of what biological and sleep research contributes and continues to clarify with respect to the SP and LD, the phenomenological world of these dreamers seeks and demands a certain set of ancient skills for its understanding and mastery.

The Skills of a "Sorcerer/Shaman"

This chapter is used as a general introduction to an empirical set of more specific techniques presented in Chapter Five. In an effort to continue to close a gap between the aesthetic, the mythical, the scientific, or the shamanic I will be using the words "sorcery" and "shamanism", broadly speaking, to mean ancient hunter-forager and shamanic practices and disciplines that scientific methodology only co-opted or thinks it has perfected. The next chapter goes into more detail regarding the actual practices and skills and the reader, if she/he would like, can go on to read that chapter and come back to this one at her/his leisure. However, there is a reason why this introduction is necessary, and the reason is an important one: it is difficult to read the sleep and dream literature comprehensively without arriving at a natural synthesis that the experiences we are talking about are "old news." Historically, dreaming "the shamanic way" has important and useful antecedents that form an important archival and experiential background for the exploration of hypnotic or meditative techniques that have an origin in these ancient practices. Both Freud and Jung saw this connection when they set out to organize and invent a science of dream interpretation and exploration. I must admit that I will fail to keep up with these two formidable minds and their scholarly syntheses in this book; but we, nevertheless, owe them a great deal and must strive to borrow the best that they can offer us.

In the context of this grander literary and scholarly field of wisdom, sometimes using the word "shaman" is more appropriate if we have reports that SP and LD dreamers utilize these skills in the context of dealing with or being "assisted" by other animal forms and entities, for example. Sometimes the word "sorcerer" would be more appropriate. Officially sanctioned or not, moreover, these practices we refer to as "socerous" or "shamanic" are also part of elaborate mystical traditions across all the major religions. However, as we shall see, for many reasons explained in earlier chapters and reasons that are pursued in the epilogue, there might also be *sound empirical reasons to focus on shamanic practices.* The often-found shamanic link in the literature of lucid dreaming attests to this appropriate and obvious inclusion. Regardless of the cultural, historical, or religious context in which these terms are found, I specifically mean all the ancient and pre-scientific empirical methods that included, and include to this day, the following principles:

1. The disciplined or routine **observation and study** of a particular phenomenon, **internal or external** to the shaman.
2. The delving into the particular "mystery" **wholeheartedly, with the totality of one's psyche and body,** as an authentic process, and sometimes despite terrifying obstacles: the risk of social or family ridicule, punishment, injury, banishment, or worse, death.
3. The hindsight design, pre-determined devising, or accidental bumping into a particular set of acts, actions, rituals; **any conjuring,** that attempts to direct, control and obtain some "grace" or favor from the phenomenon observed and its continued exploration and testing.

4.   **Transcending** the initial facts and details of—as well as internalizing and automatizing the acts, rituals; any conjuring—the phenomenon in order to reach a higher humanity, or understanding of self and universal motifs. This principle of transcendence includes the understanding of general principles and lawful processes which most organisms know only as particulars.

In these enterprises, and by abiding by these four principles, a devoted scientist and the proficient shaman see eye to eye. Thus, this SP experiencer and scientist feels quite comfortable borrowing any results and practices that derive from these sound and holistic principles.

The average SP sufferer/experiencer, as scientist or private lonely shaman, after years of being accosted by the regularity of his/her "Big" dreams, is forced into and becomes, a "sorcerer" of sorts. Assuming that the SP/LD experiences are taken to be indicators of shamanic potential in cultures worldwide, and because these "Big" dreams can occur spontaneously without the use of hallucinogenic agents, or trance-inducing exercises, they may also share elements of transcendence common to both. In the words of Michael Harner again:

"His experiences (the shaman's) are like dreams, but waking ones that feel real and in which he can control his actions and direct his adventures. While in the SSC (Shamanic State of Consciousness), he is often amazed by the reality of what is presented. He gains access to a whole new, and yet familiarly ancient universe that provides him with profound information about the meaning of his own life and death and his place within the totality of all existence. During his great adventures in the SSC, he maintains conscious control over the direction of his travels, but does not know what he will discover. He is a self-reliant explorer of the endless mansions of a magnificent hidden universe."

The alternative to "great adventures," that is, being catapulted and frozen into a situation where these four principles are not practiced at will, could lead to the situation of the frightened sufferer, a dysfunctional aspect of SP. This dysfunction may be a temporary condition or a permanent and recurring sense of powerlessness. A percentage of SP sufferers end up seeking pharmacological or clinical help in order to abate, minimize or even eradicate the SP experience altogether. For them, for religious or personal reasons, the phenomenology of the SP experience is an attack on what they believe in and can control and they would do anything to make it go away. Who wouldn't, when what is allowed to be ordinary or normal consciousness excludes these experiences and passes negative judgment on their function? This dysfunction, transient or permanent, could translate, according to my own experiences and according to the narratives shared by so many, into the following:

1. Initial (temporary) or long-term social isolation
2. Social anxiety, paranoia, or anxious behavior
3. Taking everyday reality to be an extension of a dreadful or half-understood dream, thus confusing inner and outer realities (our earlier scenarios where the dream-as-a-poem is misinterpreted)
4. Being emotionally dependant on an external, unauthentic, partial, one-dimensional, un-ecological, support source or explanation
5. Marital misunderstanding, discord, familial discord
6. Frustration, depression or even apathy in finding that cherished belief systems are not enough to offset or prevent the incidence of these mostly nocturnal events
7. Reliance on supernatural explanations for the phenomenon at the exclusion or expense of psychological explanations.

The shaman-dreamer usually experiences one or several of these negative situations before it dawns on him/her to take control and command of these experiences along testable and edifying paths. Furthermore, the literature on shamanism lists one or more of these dysfunctions as a specific call to the shamanic life. For example, the renowned historian of the shamanic, Mircea Eliade in his *Rites and Symbols of Initiation* (1958) writes about this distressing situation as follows:

"A common experience of the call to shamanism is a psychic or spiritual crisis, which often accompanies a physical or even a medical crisis, and is cured by the shaman him or herself . . . The shaman is often marked by eccentric behavior such as periods of melancholy, solitude, visions, singing in his or her sleep, etc. The inability of the traditional remedies to cure the condition of the shamanic candidate and the eventual self cure by the new shaman is a significant episode in development of the shaman. The underlying significant aspect of this experience, when it is present, is the ability of the shaman to manage and resolve periods of distress."

The next chapter provides what I believe to be a sensible way out of this situation when sleep paralysis is at the center of the psychic turmoil. As in Eliade's passage, these techniques are proposed to empower the dreamer, to make the experiencer himself/herself the central agent of well being through a path of self-discovery. Also, these techniques, although they have modern terms, truly belong to the ancient (and contemporary) world of shamanic experience. Before we go to that chapter, in the next section I will focus on a handful of common uncanny experiences, in addition to sleep paralysis itself, that if not dealt with adequately can lead to the dysfunctional outcomes outlined above: the frightened sufferer. As examples of and an overlap between the SP/LD and shamanic experiences in general, I have selected from Appendix I the following dream or dream-related experiences which occur independently from a traditional and deliberate shamanic life or practice and across cultures where these experiences may be known, dealt with, or seized for personal advancement. I will quickly go over the following experiences: hypnogogic hallucinations, nightmares, flying, OBEs, and the experiences of going through tunnels. This short list and discussion excludes something more important: the patterns of information that result from these experiences.

Specific Links Between SP, LD and Shamanic Journeys: What the "Shaman" Faces

Under unusual conditions, and as part of the rituals of preparing to go to sleep, subjects have reported what they referred to as visions, which occur when they knew that they were not asleep. Because these events are rarely mentioned in the dream literature as dreams per se[54], all I can offer here is a personal account and hope that other lucid dreamers can relate. I feel that in the context of my frequent and unusual experiences with SP, I am obligated to report this event as well as belonging to perhaps a larger continuum of related experiences.

One afternoon in 1984, after a year of more intense Zazen meditation (three times a day), adhering to a vegetarian regime and fasting[55], I laid down to rest on my living room couch without feeling the least bit tired nor intending to take a nap. I remember being very calm and rested looking at the ceiling, the walls, in a no-thought kind of mental state. Then, I simply closed my eyelids, as if in an automatic act between saccades, when, suddenly, upon opening them, my living room had disappeared except for the couch (and me upon it). Instead of walls and ceilings, a gigantic tunnel made of gently circling clouds against a tubular blue sky gyrated. Of course, my first inclination was to panic but I was equally fascinated by the spectacle before my eyes. I noticed the couch with me upon it entering the tunnel through its middle surrounded by clouds and skies in this tubular fashion, clouds that must have been miles away on top, beneath and all around me. Other than giving rise to a very tranquil state, the tunnel was not beckoning me to enter it further; it was just there. I took glances of everything within my field of vision. The details of the cloud formation, my hands, the fabric of the couch were all as distinct and "mundane" as any cloud, hand, or fabric I had ever seen; the only difference was that the context was surreal. This was a fully integrated reality and state of consciousness.

Then, I closed my eyelids, also in an autonomic response, and immediately I found myself in familiar surroundings once again. The whole experience felt phasic, as though I had gone from one reality frame into another, without missing a beat, without experiencing anything unusual between these cognitive or conscious frames. One second my eyes were open and looking into familiar surroundings, then they flickered and opened again, looking at a tubular formation of sky and clouds, then they flickered and I was back where I started. I got up from the couch very excited, finally calmed down and decided, consistent with Zen literature, that I had experienced one of those "annoying" distractions, an obstacle to mature meditation practice. The whole episode lasted less than a minute. For the record, I was not taking any drugs that could account for this event, and, in fact, at the time I was in complete opposition to their use given the path I was following.

It is at least interesting, and might even be relevant, that the above hypnogogic experience includes a worldwide shamanic preoccupation with tunnels, spinning, earth apertures, journeys through openings, and similar motifs. Entering these apertures is induced and then controlled by the shaman as a way to enter mythical lower and underworlds. One can say that Zen meditation, under the extreme circumstances in which I was practicing, was a sort of shamanic ritual, or that the various forms of meditation are derivatives of shamanic practice (although I did not think about my practice in those terms then).

In conjunction with, and as a result of entering the mystical or mythical openings, the feeling of flying is also part of these overlapping experiences, shamanic journeys and SP/LD events. Specific to the SP experience, flying sometimes occurs when an SP experiencer gains control of his/her paralysis condition and wills "flying" from the belly area. In such cases, the SP experiencer may first experience feeling compressed, or squeezed through a tunnel space, cavities, or ribbons before she/he can "fly". Variations of actual dream flying include experiences of gliding, floating, rising gently, walking or running effortlessly in big leaps[56].

As mentioned before, while in the grip of SP, it is sometimes possible to spontaneously or by choice, "wriggle out" of the paralysis by means of pushing, traveling, or crawling through a tight space usually reported as a tunnel or a corridor. These sensations may be parsimoniously explained as going to sleep in tight clothing, or sleeping while tightly wrapped in sheets or sleeping bags. *But whatever causes the initial association between the sleeping condition and the beginning of a shamanic journey, the extrusion of one's own body arrives as a logical and cognitive solution while in dream lucidity: I was trapped, I wriggled my way out that paralysis, and now I exist outside my body with/in another body. What one does afterwards with the reemergence of a body image in dream lucidity is another sort of conjuring.*

The SPS methodology reported in the next chapter includes remembering that while in SP one can divert one's attention to an area of the body typically, the navel region, in order to purposely experience the spinning and going through the tunnel. This sensation is not unlike the feeling of being sucked into and at the same time shrunk or made flexible in order to fit through a tunnel. The similarities between the SP/LD experiences and the shamanic journey can be seen when one reads anthropologist Michael Harner. For example, he says, "Entrances into the Lowerworld commonly lead down into a tunnel or tube that conveys the shaman to an exit, which opens out upon bright and marvelous landscapes." He specifically cites the experiences of an Iglulik shaman as, "He almost glides as if falling through a tube so fitted to his body that he can check his progress by pressing against the sides," or the account of a Tavgi Samoyed shaman, "As I looked around, I noticed a hole in the earth . . . The hole became larger and larger. We descended through it and arrived at a river with two streams flowing in opposite directions."

The Nightmare

Unfortunately for the dream researcher, the term nightmare is both *a dream type* and *a negative emotional qualifier* for other dream events to the extent that most people use the term to refer to a very bad and intense dream (the same duality and ambiguity occurs with the Spanish term *Pesadilla*). In this sense, the term nightmare is very imprecise for a scientific study unless it can be operationalized and given a universal sign meaning: either bad dream or SP specific. Folkloric studies of SP need to begin with attention to any anthropological keyword reference to "bad dreams" or "evil dreams" because it may be the case that field investigators generically translate these as nightmares. In my ten-year report I refer to nightmares as Negative Content dreams, which are different from hypnogogic or hypnopompic hallucinations such as the incubus. Elsewhere in the literature, as Hufford observes, nightmares are of two types. One is associated with the SP experience and usually includes a hypnogogic hallucination. This experience is identical to the older definition and experience of nightmare, or incubus. In such cases there might be an actual attack by a singular entity or a variety of beings, actual touching be unseen hands, or even the feeling of a sinister entity or presence (FOP) lurking about in the bedroom. I encourage the reader to read David Hufford's more complete elaboration of the complexity of what we English speakers refer to as a nightmare, and of its particular use as a term when referring to SPs. In short, this apparently understood word needs to be qualified when doing SP research and differentiated from simply a 'bad' or a 'negative content' dream, from sleep paralysis, from an experience of a sensed presence (FOP), and from sleep paralysis with an incubus.

Out-of-body Experiences

An out-of-body experience, OBE, is the cognitive realization that there is a sort of dream-body that exists independently of the sleeping, physical body. This is confirmed when the experiencer sometimes "sees" his/her physical body lying in his/her bed while he/she floats about in the bedroom (Blackmore, 1982; 1984). As we read in Ms. Gillis' narrative and in my own report of an OBE, the dreaming body interacts with its physical analog or other items, usually in the dreamer's own bedroom. Additional confirmation comes when the dreamer "bumps" into objects or looks at very fine details of objects and textures thought to be present in the bedroom. This exploration of one's surroundings and realization occurs with intense self-awareness, which itself leads to curiosity and the further study of how to operate in this state. As reported in the text, OBEs can and do occur sometimes in conjunction with the very first SP experience and in subsequent events. During the ten years of official recording of SP episodes there were four OBEs that occurred in the same night as an SP event, either preceding an SP event, or following it. Equally, an OBE experience can turn into flying, gliding, standing, dragging oneself on the ground with great effort, floating, or rising gently. Interestingly, OBEs are rarely about walking and have an affinity to both the "flying" experiences of LD and the paralysis often cited in reports as a feeling of being glued, or stuck to a certain spot in the dreamer's room. That is, OBEs can also be expressed as part of the SP experience since the dreaming body gets stuck too!

Finally, the use of trance states, hypnosis, self-hypnosis, and meditation are elements of shamanic practices. The next chapter introduces both self-hypnosis and meditation as aspects of SPS, as modern shamanic tools for controlling the dream circumstances we have been describing. It is with the volitional and purposeful deployment of these techniques that the SP sufferer can move from a potentially dysfunctional situation one cannot interpret, react to, or control to a "shamanic" LD and more positive journey and exploration.

The next section introduces a visual aid and model that maps the above states in a convenient and simple way. This very image and model may be instructive to a person who is only beginning to understand, and cannot classify, internal states, much less the various dreaming states. This map is also a first step, an empirical shamanic device, on the way to conjuring or controlling lucid dreaming that ensues from the SP experience.

The Dreaming Cube: A Sorcerous/Shamanic Map

Earlier we sketched out Hobson's and MacCarly's Activation Synthesis dream bio-psychological model and decided with others (LaBerge, in particular, 1985; 2000) that it is a correct observation of what happens at hind, mid and forebrain cerebral levels when we enter into REM states, but that it has psychological limitations when it comes to understanding the reemergence, not only of self-awareness in dreaming, but of control of dream psychological states. More strongly put, LaBerge (2000) raises the bar on proposals that aim to describe dreaming without accounting for lucid states when he says:

"Theories of dreaming that do not account for lucidity are incomplete, and theories that do not allow for lucidity are incorrect.[57]*"*

I agree with LaBerge's strong challenge both from the perspective of an SP/LD experiencer and a sleep researcher, but being a thrifty person and an open-minded explorer I will nevertheless borrow wisdom when I see it even from an incomplete model. The "sorcerer" or the "shaman" is a pragmatic being.

That means that the model presented in this chapter is also inspired by Hobson's own AIM[58] model for identifying normal and dysfunctional psychological states. I modeled the *shamanic dream cube* after his, partly to include a demonstration of an alternative existential-cognitive interpretation, and also because I believe that, once again, sometime in the future, when LaBerge's concerns have been addressed, and the bio-psychology is solid, it could be used as a springboard to explain higher order levels of cerebral functioning in a way that satisfies an ecologically complex phenomenon. In other words, Hobson's is a bio-psychological model and cube, mine is more existential-cognitive, but both could be overlapped and translated into one another whenever needed when psychological science catches up to both. More importantly, the shamanic model presented here may serve as a heuristic and a call to expand Hobson's AIM model in sleep research to finally include self-aware lucidity.

Although a bit simplistic even by Hobson's own admission, I nevertheless find AIM to be a powerful and elegant illustration and model for consciousness. Our dreaming cube, because it borrows from Hobson's, is also simplistic because it aims to capture a vast continuum of dream consciousness in a simply model. But, secretly, I hope that other psychology-shaman-scientists, when reading about the kind of widespread work that their minds and mind products give rise to, will be more embracing of these efforts and contribute their amazing talents to an infinitely more difficult task: the interdisciplinary approach. With all these talents at hand the cube may be expanded into more refined reincarnations and uses.

So then, as a way of attempting a common language among specialist dream researchers and psychologists alike, and for empirical purposes, it was helpful to me to quantify and scale dream events, types and categories (Appendix I) along a phenomenological continuum, from a no-dream situation, through *flimsies* (see also Appendix I), then *regular dreams*, followed by *vivid dreams*, continuing on to *extra vivid dreams*, followed by *lucid dreams*, *sleep paralysis*, and this continuum ending in a hypnogogic experience that is perceived to be REAL (as the one shared earlier in this chapter). *This scale might be useful to the scientist as shaman, but it is indispensable to the dreamer-shaman as a basic general map of his/her own consciousness while dreaming.* To put the map to a test, and as Figure 2 illustrates, SP and LD experiences are localizable on a four-dimensional map of consciousness, our shamanic dreaming cube, that includes virtual and real behavioral, perceptual, affective, and cognitive states. The increased intensities along these four experiential dimensions (coded as "+" or "-" signs) contribute to and are summed up in a fifth dimension: *the overall degree of vividness or lucidity or even of self-awareness.* For the purposes of simplifying an already complex figure I have combined functionality and perception under one axis.

Figure 2: Dreaming Cube

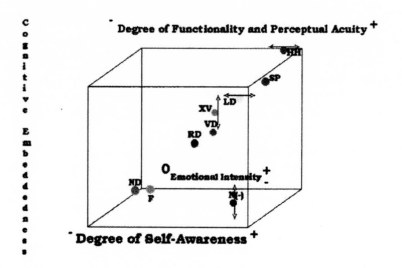

Figure 2, A Dreaming Cube Map—The dreaming cube is a three-dimensional representation and a way of illustrating the phenomenological quality of any dream experience. Given the values indicated by the subject dream report and index (Appendix IV) any dream experience—or its absence—can be categorized according to a *Functional Control, Perceptual Acuity, Intensity of Emotion*, and *Cognitive Embeddedness* dimension. Thus the *vividness* of a dream event—or the absence of a dream—is the general and summed evaluation of the interaction of these dimensions. In this figure a lucid dream, LD, ranks high on cognitive embeddedness, degree of self-awareness and degree of *functionality* and *perceptual acuity* whereas a "flimsy," F, ranks low on all these dimensions. For the purposes of simplicity I have combined the values of *Functional Control* and *Perceptual Acuity*. Finally, this figure illustrates *Intensity of Emotion* as well as its valences: positive or negative.

To further illustrate, within the space of this cube and model, one can operationalize dream types and the dream/sleep phenomenological continuum and further specify "vividness" (also implied in the intensity of self-awareness) in terms of:

1) Degrees of *functional control* (body movements, sleep paralysis[59], walking, eating, meditating, talking, flying, etc.)

2) *Perceptual acuity* (black and white-to-color, texture, face discrimination-identification, blurry images to sharp colored scenes)

3) The *intensity of the emotion* felt, or its valence, positive or negative[60].

4) A cognitive dimension, *cognitive embeddedness*, that specifies the *quality and degree of information obtained* while involved in any dream event. This last dimension is significant to the SP and LD experiences when one considers, for example, the type of exchanges that occurred in the lucid and recurrent dream I related earlier in Chapter Three. Actual information gathering and practical gains within or outside the lucid dreamscape corroborate this interpretative dimension as an important example of the continuity of all consciousness-with-self-awareness, a point on which I will elaborate further in the last section of this chapter.

So, the *vividness* of a dream event, as reported by many authors including myself, found in my dream event classification in all published reports, is a more general category (or more precisely, a semiotic *code—a complex of cognitive-semantic functions*) that combines *self-awareness, functionality, perceptual acuity, degree of emotion* felt, and *cognitive embeddedness*. Furthermore, I believe these dimensions to be adequate in capturing most events described in dream content work, shamanic experience, and laboratory methodology and classification even if improvements can be made. My claim here is that this shamanic model is sufficient to begin talking about a shamanic journey, when the shamanic journey involves SP/LD experiences, that it has a pragmatic value. Its validity is secure to the extent that the four dimensions reflect minimum and realistic experiential parameters that are easily recognizable by the SP/LD experiencer or average dreamer alike. These parameters can then be translated to pursue the many faces and cross-cultural versions of the SP/LD experience with a common empirical ground and tool.

Additionally, I am confident that these dimensions and their more specific constructs can be turned into paper and pencil forms to record and further specify dreams along these or additional dimensions. Short of that, these recorded experiences can be scored and illustrated afterwards by using what I call a *Dreaming Reality Index* (see Appendix IV) that can be graphed in a cube such as the one shown in Figure 2. By the way, in case the reader is wondering how I arrived at the specific x,y,z placements, I simply assigned purely arbitrary increments to Dream Events (Type or Category) using a Fibonacci number series.[61] Although a subjective tool, in addition to including basic dream events found in dream content surveys and questionnaires research, it improves these by attempting a gradation, to scale, of the degree to which a dreamer is more, less, or not at all "found" in these consciousness spaces.

Relevant to the states of consciousness depicted in the dreaming cube, and as Austin (1999) indicates, it is possible to identify dozens if not hundreds of consciousness states that extend beyond the dreaming experience and overlap with other states such as meditation, hypnosis, and even being awake[62]. For the purposes of this writing the presentation of the shaman map or cube is an attempt at drawing basic distinctions between SP, LD, and other dream events and expanding the AIM model to include every sort of consciousness event conceivable, if this is even possible.

The dreaming cube is therefore a map of dream phenomenology that serves the purpose of sighting and tracking self-awareness and consciousness. As we said before, it has the advantage that, unlike Hobson's AIM psychochemical model, it is psychologically open ended so that even when psychochemical findings can be added later that may explain the coordinates and positions, the phenomenology of the dreamer figures more prominently than the neurochemistry. It is ultimately a subjective tool that, bypassing the developing biological story, can be used off the shelf so-to-speak to assist the "shaman" or to attempt a psychological unity between his/her dreaming and waking lives. I will seek further synthesis by addressing one more time, in different words, the point that in addition to arguing that maintaining a psychological unity is an essential aspect of wellness, this unity is itself maintained in raw consciousness when humans do not impose artificial boundaries.

Finally, a portion of the dreaming cube can be tested mathematically and visually by approaching the nature of self-aware consciousness using a fractal model by differentiating between at least five types of consciousness states and/or dream phenomenology: 1-awake consciousness; 2-no dreams, 3-regular dreams, 4-vivid dreams; and 5-lucid dreams or dreams with consciousness. The portion of the dreaming cube that can be tested would be the continuity of self-awareness that span from awake to lucid dreaming states. More clearly, the idea would be to *delineate self-awareness wherever it appears in conscious states distinguishing it from states of consciousness that lack self-awareness*. More specifically, thorough the use of Mandelbrot and/or Julia sets and the numerical results of the pencil-and-paper questionnaire tool for assessing dream lucidity described earlier, one could accomplish the following:

1) Label and distinguish between consciousness with self-awareness (present in awake and lucid dreams) as ORDER states and non-consciousness as CHAOS.

2) Distinguish the smallest boundary between ORDER and CHAOS in a precisely defined continuum of consciousness and dream phenomenology where ORDER is always represented by increases in self-awareness.

3) Show in pictorial and mathematical formats that "self-similarity" occurs between awake consciousness and lucid dreams or dreams with consciousness.

4) Be able to translate and plug in the numbers one obtains from this measure of dream consciousness with lucidity—self-awareness—into Mandelbrot and/or Julia sets in order to iterate until it can be shown that lucid dreaming "belongs" to a "lucidity" set and not outside it.

In short, and in keeping to contributions of other ideas of the fractalization of mind states, cognitive information and neuronal events[63], I wonder if it is possible to extend the idea of fractal modularity to also include or mean *Meta-fractal-modularity, a coarse and metaphorical boundary of the many forms of conscious lucidity.*

This exploration in another fashion, of the continuity of consciousness with self-awareness, is precisely the focus of the next section.

The Unity and the Extension of Consciousness

As a way of putting together the many threads developed in this chapter and throughout this book, it is worth revisiting and further establishing a premise that unites all these themes. The premise is that consciousness, as Austin and others aptly have realized, incorporates a larger continuum of experiences even though it appears,[64] phenomenologically speaking, that there is discontinuity of mental states. One apparent discontinuity in the west is that between normal and altered states of consciousness. But on the other hand, we all accept that when we are tired and fatigued, or when we are engaged in daydreaming, all these states, although different from being perky-awake and alert, are part of a GRANDER consciousness we deem unitary. If so, then a psychological proposal that presents consciousness vaguely, or incomplete proposals of what consciousness is or is not, originating mainly within a modern western culture, are limiting noetic exercises because, in reality, consciousness exists as a vast continuum of human experiences for many cultures and times. The cherishing of nature as the source of the "spiritual" and the continuity of nature into an ecological conscious and unconscious that we demote to an inferior cognitive status, that of animism, is nevertheless, evidence that consciousness was perceived by ancients to be if not seamless, at least continuous and interacting with its many layers.

So the complexity and continuity of consciousness, even when refused and ignored by dogma or law, even when we have forgotten what to do in (during) the transitions between these other states, is nevertheless safely and securely represented in the experiences of other cultures or individuals who wish to expand their noetic horizons. The simplistic and debatable classification of these experiences into a consciousness-side and altered-states-of-consciousness side, sets limits to what "normal" consciousness could be about, and at the same time, reduces the other side of this dubious dichotomy to something less than an ideal sort of mental state.

To borrow and then re-apply a wonderful sentence I quoted earlier from Harner, if the purpose of consciousness is to serve "a self-reliant explorer of the endless mansions of a magnificent hidden universe," then the scope of consciousness itself needs to be rediscovered and expanded to include all of the mansions within and their interactions with the natural world; the ultimate source of who we are. Specific to the shamanic experience Dr. Benny Shannon (2003)[65] writes:

"The dynamic nature of consciousness should be borne in mind. Consciousness is a system that spans an entire range of possibilities along which, at different times, different profiles emerge. Throughout our lives, the values associated with the parameters of the system consciousness are constantly changing. The values in dreaming differ from those in normal wakefulness, those encountered when we are fresh and alert differ from those encountered in fatigue, and all these differ from those exhibited in the extreme states usually referred to as 'altered (or alternate) states of consciousness.' Since consciousness is always changing, always alternating, the term 'altered/alternate states of consciousness' is, I find, deceptive."

Shanon proposes a theoretic reformulation of consciousness where it can be "defined by a set of parameters that can take different values." He writes that his statement is in opposition to William James' presentation of consciousness as consisting of a more exclusive or restrictive "set of features." To the extent that these features are defined and prescribed by a western mind that can be seen as MIND-bankrupt or that fears the open-ended consciousness of dream lucidity, it is understandable that it belittles, demotes, and under-represents its aesthetic possibilities. On the other hand, the dreaming cube suggests that the parameter "self-awareness," if one argues that this is definitional of consciousness, takes on different "values" between awake and sleep states in a cyclical fashion with respect to those individuals who dream lucidly. If consciousness is defined by yet another parameter, "bounded-by-the-idea-of-a-body," then consciousness so defined is equally cyclical between awake and sleep states in the lucid dreamer. The lucid dreamer can project a dreaming body, or not, but this freedom is not even an option for the physical body during awake consciousness. But even when we adhere to a more orthodox account of consciousness, the lucid dreamer is more awake than asleep; therefore his/her explorations need to be investigated more seriously because now they have entered the realm of waking phenomenology.

If a complete understanding of consciousness still depends on an explanation of dream lucidity, then philosophers or psychologists who demote and oversimplify dreaming to a footnote about "the dream experience" as an exception to a certain rational-when-awake rule (in order to be dismissed from a grandiose consciousness-explained scheme of their own invention) are surely on shaky ground simply because their theory is non-inclusive.

To reiterate an earlier point, if aesthetics endures beyond the awake state into dreaming-with-volition, and aesthetics is a purposeful enterprise, then the aesthetic products that result from SP/LD dreaming are as important as the ones obtained and explored during the awake states, or any other state for that matter. Once again, Shanon seems to be in agreement with my proposal when he refers to the shamanic journey resulting from taking the hallucinogen ayahuasca when he says:

"The phenomenology of the ayahuasca experience suggests that within the definition of human consciousness exist some parameters that are not part of regular contemporary discourse. I refer to the parameters of aesthetics and sanctity. I propose that these are basic determinants of human cognition; correspondingly, they might be grounded in the very structure of the brain."

Shanon's claim is all the more reassuring not only because it echoes the case I have already made for revisiting aesthetics as a undercurrent for the mythical, the shamanic or SP/LD dreaming, but because he finds it so fundamental to a definition of consciousness. The aesthetic component of consciousness is part of his "semantic parameters" or what I have been referring to the semiosis of dreaming. Because this aesthetic element can be that much richer and informative during psychedelic or SP/LD experiences then, it is attended to with fuller and greater consciousness, and thus new meaning is not only derived, but also expanded and created. The aesthetic experience itself can move seamlessly into the mystical experience. I ask once again my now tiring question: If mainstream aesthetics is valued and written about, and mystically produced aesthetics is valued and written about, and even if the hallucinogenic-shamanic experience is valued and written about, then why should a potent and naturally induced state of conscious lucidity and derived aesthetics be any less valuable than any of the other states and products?

Equally, Shanon makes a distinction I made earlier, while reviewing Langer's view of aesthetics between an actual meaningful and purposeful experience and disorganized, psychotic, mental products. To him the experiences of the shaman are "well-structured and laden with meaning whereas those of the psychotic are often fragmentary and chaotic." If this distinction worked for Langer, and works for Shanon, then by logical extension, IT MUST BE APPLIED to the SP/LD experience as well.

If purposeful, non-chaotic mental operations are one of the measures by which we could assign a higher "production" quality or value to consciousness, then the non-ordinary and willed SP/LD experience of a sober lucid dreamer is at least on equal footing as the willed journey of the shaman who ingests ayahuaska. More strongly, I will argue with the religious traditions that employ meditation as a vehicle into the uncanny that in fact the SP/LD experience is that much more pure or honest because it requires no pharmaceutical props and because it has a longer and more pervasive influence on the day to day life of the "shaman."[66]

Of course, to be naturally endowed to the shamanic is not the same as force-feeding the mythical with botanicals, but since they both share important visual and experiential elements, shouldn't we study in-depth the naturally occurring phenomenon with the same interest and scientific curiosity? It may not be the case as some authors have suggested that ingestion of mind-enhancing botanicals gave rise to the mythical and/or the mystical, but rather that a handful of individuals have always existed who tapped into these states regardless of whether or not they could find that "god herb" of magic mushroom. As we argued earlier, it might have been (and still is) beneficial to our species to have had a small but consistent population of dreamers possessing dreaming capabilities with a wider ranging cognitive scope that could generate ideas, concepts and other adaptations required for survival. This line of thinking takes me to the realm of speculation and compels me to ask: Can narcolepsy itself be the dysfunctional dual inheritance of a dream-lucidity genetic code that when only partially expressed gives rise to the SP/LD dreamer? As a way of an analogy, and as in the case of sickle-cell anemia, narcolepsy is disadvantageous for sure when a dual genetic representation occurs, but the singular SP/LD inheritance confers a useful adaptation: open-ended creative dreaming. Forgive me, these are stray thoughts that I will need to explore elsewhere.

To close this chapter, even Shanon, willing to as he is expand the construct of consciousness so the ayahuaska induced shamanic experience has a credible place in the firmament of what is accepted in western psychology and philosophy, oversimplifies dreaming. For example, when talking about the ability of the hallucinogen ayahuaska to enhance reality he says, "Dreams and imagination usually decrease the value assigned to this parameter [The conferral of reality]; the ayahuaska experience may increase it."

Only lucid dreamers know for sure and are qualified to talk about their "Big" dreams, and only lucid dreamers are in a position to evaluate the affinity that their experience has with other reported phenomena and their full experiential integration with the whole of consciousness. All together, whether we know it or not, the inebriated shamans, sober shamans, artists who pretend to be shamans, philosophers of consciousness who wish to be shamans, alien-abductees who should be on shamanic journeys, are converging on a similar *noesis*: the mythical. One can only ignore mythos at one's own psychological peril.

The next chapter thus, is an opportunity to share with you, reader and practitioner of the uncanny, a set of information ('conjuring' and 'incantations') that aims at assisting in this converging toward *noesis*. They are preliminary steps, but important, foundational steps, in beginning to unite uncanny and wakeful consciousness in a healthy way.

The skills of the shaman outlined at the beginning of this chapter, include the practical and empirical conjuring expanded in Chapter Five. But in keeping with Shannon's sentiments and thesis, one must not lose sight of the final aim, a moving developmental target, toward transcending the very steps we take to make coherent the dual and accelerated contributions of both discursive and non-discursive realities.

I think *poesis* is a temporary form of **transcendence** at first if one is, like me, trained as an objective, linear thinking scientist. This movement expands consciousness. However, true **transcendence**, I think, is moving beyond poesis AND a rational outlook. But I am not there yet; I continue to vacillate between one and the other, each swing providing fodder and sustenance to the other **noetic** side. I don't know how many developmental 'swings' it takes to make a psyche whole. This is the path toward Individuation that Jung spoke about, the reuniting of all psychic parts into a complete Self. If so, *poesis* represents female or anima and the rational outlook the male or the animus. The final reunion of these two aspects of being may be an impossible task, but pursuing their interplay is more than knowing what is going on in one's own mental house. It is even more than seeking a reality that is, as Shannon said earlier, "well-structured and laden with meaning" away from the risk of a "psychotic . . . fragmentary and chaotic" psychological makeup.

I agree with Jung and other humanist psychologists that being on the path toward whatever form of ***transcendence*** we are capable of, given our finite time on this planet and psychological limitations, is necessary for well being. If so, then the journey I have been sharing with you, because it is imposed by my biology, demands that much attention.

We don't all have to be uncanny dreamers to derive some personal benefit from this journey. If we are open to the stories of others, we can be impacted and grow and appreciate the products of this journey as art forms and personal philosophy. I have been made anew by the voices, the stories, the songs, and the journeys of people whose experiences are and will be beyond my experiential reach. An additional perspective in life is as good as gold. So now you also know that scientists can be 'shamans.'

At the very least you can understand why is it that I am crankier than the next person, some say, easily frustrated by the superficial, the material, the waste of time protecting false personas. You can understand at least why I seek nature as medicine, and defend nature from greedy hands. Some of the mythical is totemic and the source of the totemic is OUT THERE in nature and also part of ME. Uncanny dreaming never lets me forget this connection; it completes a psychic circle that is about FULL consciousness. One can only ignore mythos at one's own psychological peril because mythos is always connected to a real composition of biological bodies embedded in Earth's GROUND.

CHAPTER FIVE

Sleep Paralysis Signaling: A Skills System for Transitioning from SP to LD

> *"Once I discovered that memory was the key to lucid dreaming, further practice and methodological refinements allowed me to arrive, within a year, at my goal: a method by which I could reliably induce lucid dreams."*
>
> Stephen LaBerge, *Lucid Dreaming: The Power of Being Awake & Aware in Your Dreams*

This chapter introduces a description, recommendation, and a set of techniques for naturally and effectively cuing lucid dreaming while in the atonic state of Isolated Sleep Paralysis (ISP). These presentations originate from the empirically tested claim that in fact sleep paralysis can be, and is, used as a powerful signaling prime and prelude to lucid dreaming. For simplicity's sake I have termed this set of maneuvers *Sleep Paralysis Signaling*, or *SPS*. Additionally, throughout this chapter I will make the argument that SP may be one of the most effective and robust natural ways for inducing lucid dreaming, superior to other methodologies discussed elsewhere. I will first describe three discernable clusters or categories of experiences that I refer to as the *three phases of cuing* that the SP experiencer can easily detect with the intact self-awareness preserved during SP. Also, two main methods for anxiety management during paralysis are described: a self-hypnotic induction and meditation. Both methods are aimed at controlling and reducing the anxiety and powerlessness associated with ISP. The case is made that the inherent awareness of these phases (and the cognitive method they give rise to), because SP must also be considered as a *hyper-mnemonic symptom*, are more accessible and less cumbersome than external devices that are commercially available for cuing Lucid Dreaming such as *DreamLight* (LaBerge, 1995) or more cognitive methods such as Mnemonic Induction (LaBerge, 1985). Even though I am the first to admit that these other methods are helpful and necessary when the SP symptomology does not exist, nevertheless the SP experiencer already has an advantage with respect to the "average" dreamer, an advantage that can be exploited if the fear associated with paralysis can be circumvented or appeased.

Additionally, I will share with the readers a widely employed hypno-therapeutical technique, *anchoring*, that can be used equally for reducing the anxiety associated with the paralysis of SP, enhancing awareness during SP, or facilitating the dreaming unfolding from SP to LD. As a way of summarizing a varied and potentially confusing list of techniques and dream phenomena I will pause midway through this chapter to write about both a theoretical and experiential rationale for the above positions.

Also important in recognizing, anticipating, and controlling dreaming are the more or less predictable phenomenological *unfolding* of pre-dormital and sleep onset sequences described at the end of this chapter. Three such sequences are categorized and described as a result of applying the "shamanic" and empirical principles described in the previous chapter. The three unfolding sequences can be taken as a bare bones description of the *SPS* phases about to be described.

Sleep Paralysis Signaling (SPS)

Throughout years of experiencing this state of *bound*

lucidity, ISP, the experiencer, if he/she does not want to control the condition through pharmacological means or counseling, has to develop less invasive, more private, and more psychological means and skills to deal with his/her condition. I, as well as 15% of the subjects who participated in the studies described in the full-length articles, have corroborated that the ISP condition, since it is concurrent with lucid dreaming in a lot of cases, can be used as a natural cue for inducing lucid dreaming akin to feedback with electronic devices such as *DreamLight* (LaBerge, 1995) that alert the dreamer at the onset of oculo-motor activity and head motion. As it is in my case, it is my hope that, barring any other serious side effects (unbearable anxiety or prolonged insomnia), the chronic sleep paralysis sufferer can turn this condition to an experiential advantage and transform *bound lucid states* into lucid dreaming.

Phenomenological Feedback: SPS Phases

Subjects who experience SP routinely are in a unique position, a position of advantage over the average lucid dreamer or infrequent enticer of these experiences, since they can exploit the paralysis situation and use it as a launch pad, so to speak, for achieving dream lucidity. *Functionally speaking, and in the context of eliciting lucid dreams, I am referring to this specific use of the sleep paralysis state to achieve these ends as Sleep Paralysis Signaling (SPS).* The phenomenological sequence used to practically and routinely cue Lucid Dreaming can be described as follows:

Phase One

Upon finding oneself in the atonic state, *a reacquisition of self-awareness,* **SPS** *includes the ability to garnish and focus one's attention on some part of the body* (focusing on the belly area works for me but other subjects report different areas) *while breathing purposely and calmly.* Without going any further with this attentional discipline, or wanting to achieve lucid dreaming, the anxiety associated with SP may pass and the subject may either wake up or begin dreaming.

Phase Two

The second phase of **SPS** includes similar techniques to those used for achieving lucid dreaming such as *imagining the body spinning with the navel area as a center, imagining being crumbled up as if a piece of paper, falling, or floating away* (and Gillis, Personal Communication). Part of this second phase includes, for this subject, something he terms the "roll up" trick. After focusing on the navel area, the paralysis eases into any of these sensations, but more strongly into the sensation that one is being curled into a ball, very tightly, and the body then disappears into the navel region. *This sensation usually precedes the experience of falling, or going through the commonly reported tunnel.*

Phase Three

At "the end of the tunnel", a third set of qualitatively different experiences awaits the dreamer. *It includes entering a lucid dream state and maintaining consciousness to the proper level of alertness so as to extend the experience of the controlled dreamscape and/or interact with dream images or beings.* The interactions with these beings are intense and subjectively real, and their full explication is outside the scope of this presentation. The ultimate constraint for the duration of this controlled experience and phase is physiological, dependent on the amount of REM sleep allotted for that particular cycle in the evening. Until someone devises a means to prolong REM sleep periods, these exotic dream episodes will remain short, sweet, and fleeting for most dreamers. Thus, throughout these three phases, consciousness is fading incrementally, from the first awareness of paralysis to the last flying dream. Nevertheless, when **SPS** is used for the specific purpose of inducing these states, then LDs and OBEs ensue and a greater degree of awareness and control of the dreaming experience is achieved.

Self-hypnosis and Meditation: Inducing Both ISPs and LDs

Self-Hypnosis—At last one report exists in the medical literature of 'treating' SP with hypnosis (Nardi, 1981). Before my training in neurocognition I was a student of hypnotherapy, and have logically employed self-hypnosis when I was aware that sleep paralysis might be commencing. I and other subjects, for example, *report odd body sensations, almost electrical, prior to experiencing SPs and coinciding with being abnormally tired or jet-lagged.* Knowing this, I decided to use a simple self-hypnotic induction to ease my fears of the anticipated experience. The induction is a combination of relaxation and attentional sequences involving imagery of a fog-like (purple) and pacifying energy source entering my body through my toes and finally engulfing me as a cocoon. As the imagery progresses, anchoring techniques are incorporated into this sequence in order to induce relaxation of muscle groups from the toes to the crown of the head. Nowadays, I only have to do this sequence as pure imagery to achieve relaxation and well being. Earlier in this practice, a few years back, practicing this particular induction employed the suggestion that if I ever experienced the paralysis I would not be afraid and I would eventually fall asleep without consciousness. These suggestions are no longer required in the imagery-only sequence since I have apparently conditioned this assumption into the process without verbal reminders. *The result of this practice is entering into the SP state with the greater confidence that I am in control of this situation and, more importantly, that I experience little or no anxiety.* In the last four years or so, this practice, and/or the meditation described in the next section, has resulted in greater consciousness-fluidity and movement between the *SPS* phases described above.

Meditation—A serendipitous event precipitated the use of meditation as a gentle transition between waking and dream paralytic states. The author seriously pursued Zazen practice for several years and toward the later part of his training, increasingly so, sleep paralysis would occur coinciding with deeper and deeper meditational states (and, I must confess, with falling asleep while meditating!). Since practicing under these circumstances was too distracting, the author ceased Zazen practice altogether. As distracting as practicing meditation under these circumstances was, nevertheless, it created the condition that now the SP experience was under some measure of control. Since that year (1986) I have incorporated a simple meditation done in bed while waiting for sleep to come. For some reason, *I have adopted the induction for those days when I think SP is likely to occur and the meditation practice I reserve as a way of purposely inducing SPs or LDs when I feel alert and rested.* For this meditation I used a concentration/attentional exercise, which entails finding a comfortable position lying prone on my back (a position reported to induce SPs to begin with) with eyes closed. Then I look into the darkness, "through" the back of my eyelids, and imagine that the darkness I perceive and the minutia of visual imperfections that accompany this sort of perception create a three-dimensional space. Additionally, I am regulating my breathing, first by starting out with deep cleansing breaths, and then by allowing a shallow, unconscious breathing to replace the first type. The same breathing is utilized during the self-hypnosis. If I persist with the meditation, unusual imagery replaces the feeling that I am seeing three-dimensional space ahead of me. *Next, the experiences of going through tunnels, squeezing through a tight opening, spinning, hearing a buzzing sound, hearing clicks and crackles, and sometimes experiencing SP let me know that I have succeeded in carrying everyday awareness into a Lucid Dream sleep state.* (Please refer to Dr. James H. Austin's *Zen and The Brain*, 1999, for a detailed and wonderful exploration of all preceding sleep-imagery-lucid dreaming dynamics.) These experiences are also concomitant with the induction exercise or with falling asleep prior to experiencing SP. To reiterate, both techniques achieve similar ends of greater relaxation, less anxiety and greater control over the unfolding events. In either case, self-hypnosis or meditation, it is possible to simply fall asleep without accomplishing the more rare lucid states.

Paralysis Itself as an *Anchoring*, Hypnotic Technique

Hypnotherapy practitioners use a technique called ***anchoring*** as way of reinforcing suggestions, posthypnotic or otherwise, as a mnemonic for activating a more positive behavior as a correction or an antagonist to bad habits or circumstances. These techniques are also widely used in the management of pain and anxiety. For example, when my wife was expecting our youngest son, during the three to four months prior to her due date, she underwent several hypnosis sessions with me. Concurrent with childbirth classes the hypnosis sessions included *a particular touch on a particular part of her body* as a signal to deploy a specific breathing sequence or in order to relax. One can think of *anchoring* as a component of a posthypnotic suggestion with the aim of physically eliciting the desired behaviors by a touch signal or procedure. In the case of an expectant couple, the birth coach is given the responsibility of generating the anchor although an anchor can be self-initiated as well. Additionally, and depending on the situation, the hypnotic subject may or may not know about this anchor. In my wife's case, all the anchors we established were overt and conscious. By touching her arm in the very spot and in the specific way we had agreed on, while she was under, to her conscious and her unconscious minds this signal-by-touch meant relaxation, or breathing faster.

The widespread use of anchoring techniques in hypnotherapy are a testament to their efficacy in post-suggestive management of a multitude of behaviors, from quitting smoking to reducing anxiety in a test situation to increased confidence. One can think of anchoring as an advanced form of mnemonics, and if so, they can expand LaBerge's invitation to use ordinary memory in LD work to include a higher level of dream sophistication and manipulation.

Because sleep paralysis itself is *hyper-mnemonic*, a *hyper-mnemonic symptom*, then it is an obvious and effective candidate for anchoring. No pun intended, sleep paralysis IS THE ANCHOR! This means that in combination with pro-active hypnotherapy or even self-hypnosis (or meditation practice, see below) SP sufferers can aim to mimic the SP state while undergoing hypnosis, and in conjunction with relaxation and behavioral suggestions, transform the paralysis into a signal (a sign in a semiotic sense) to move beyond that point into the dreaming sequence.

I also suggested to one of our contributors who was already working with a willing hypnotherapist to follow (combine) the sleep-paralysis-as-an-anchor technique with a practiced, rotation of the body while under hypnosis, as if she was "water draining down a tunnel." So in her visualization, her feet went "down the drain" first. But I also suggested that this work might be accomplished in two ways. I suggested that her hypnotherapist ask her to stand up from a sitting position AFTER she had secured and practiced sleep paralysis as an anchor, slowly rotating her body with arms extended or withdrawn while flexing her knees as if she was actually being sucked or pulled down by a drain hole. Depending on one's age or the health of one's knees, this may not work (it worked for this particular subject). So instead of asking the client to stand up, she could remain on the couch or chair, "visualizing" her body rotating with the navel as a pivot until the body shrinks, flexes, or folds, moving then into a tunnel. The subject in question wrote me months later and reported great success with this technique although, as she says, "I still get stuck once in awhile." I do too!

In retrospect, as obvious as it may seem to use SP itself as the hyper-mnemonic anchor, I only stumbled on it by accident around the same time my wife was employing these techniques in order to facilitate her labor and to empower the soon-to-be birthing mother.

As I mentioned earlier, this was almost seventeen years ago when I was ending my Zazen practice and while in meditation I would freeze up in sleep paralysis! While I talked to our abbot about this, his help and suggestions did not diminish the paralysis-while-in-meditation. So next time the paralysis happened, I made it part of my technique to continue practicing my breathing and placing the totality of my attention on my navel area. Although the paralysis did not stop from recurring in my practice, and I eventually gave up Zazen, henceforth whenever SP overcame me I practiced "Zazen dreaming" and moved into LD! During these last seventeen years I have also reinforced this practice with self-hypnosis. "It works, it works, it works." I can't say it enough because if there is one technique that health practitioners can assist the SP/LD dreamer with on their way to self-growth, it is this one. I will let you discover what happens next when you become an accomplished meditator in dream space.

Rationale For SPS

Now is the time to put on my scholarly hat once again and consider grander themes and arguments. In addition to the practical considerations reviewed in the past sections, there are logical reasons why the ISP experience and events can be thought of as a natural cuing conducive to Lucid Dreaming. With practice and some discipline, a natural increment of self-awareness can be used for more creative dreaming ends. Some of the reasons for thinking so are:

1) *The atonic state itself intensifies consciousness/awareness, more so than the average lucid dream experience; it precedes it in a dreaming sequence, since now the challenge of body paralysis and waking from it is a dire issue and even a desperate act.* Regardless of whether **SPS** is pursued in a disciplined manner, or spontaneously achieved, *even this anxious state is an increment of consciousness as self-awareness.*

2) Having used the paralysis as a *hyper-mnemonic symptom*, as an anchoring device, and having conquered the paralysis by any number of disciplined attentional exercises (also disciplining the attention gained by naturally occurring paralysis) and controlled breathing, *the dreamer gains greater confidence in exploring his/her conscious/lucid dreaming condition (a positive feedback effect).*

3) Pursuing further control of a *dreaming-body image or representation* that is already easily fabricated by the naturally occurring paralysis *encourages using this image to "move" within the dreamscape.* There is a second opportunity for positive feedback loops with regard to maintaining a conscious state in the sense that *acquiring a so-called "dreaming body" enhances the illusion of mobility and thus control.* (A flying dream may be another example of this: If I am flying in my dream I must have a "body" to fly with. If I have a body to fly with, then I must be able to control that body.)

4) For the chronic sufferer of SP, inducing lucid dreams is a matter of waiting for the next bout, or series of natural SPs to occur: their anchor and a *hyper-mnemonic.*

*The very knowledge that another SP event will occur, and that all one has to do is use it as a signal to achieve LDs (through **SPS**), psychologically primes or predisposes the subject to look forward to these events, thinking that each time the fear is lessened and the control is greater.*

To be fair, **SPS** only increases the probability that SP will produce more positive outcomes than its more commonly reported anxiety, fear, or terror. Depending on the psychological state of the individual, any spontaneous SP can result in these more negative conditions without the possibility of remembering or practicing the entire **SPS** sequence. Something else needs to be in place prior to entering the sleep states that will increase the probability of entering the SP condition in an already calm and regulated psychological attitude. Also, as we said earlier, and contrary to popular LD lore, REM sleep is biologically determined and timed, so even though psychological time is distorted and it feels as though the dreamer has spent hours "flying" around, the REM clock is thoroughly objective and brings the "shaman" out only when the neurons want it unless, of course, these states can be prolonged by pharmaceutical or other means.

The Unfolding of SP and LD: Three Typical Phenomenological SP-to-LD Sequences

In Chapter Four I summarized four "shamanic" or empirical principles of transcendence (in our case transcending the limitations and the fright associated with SP per se) that I claimed are basic empirical attitudes and methodologies necessary for *stalking the uncanny*. By applying these principles other dreamers and myself have observed the following sequences leading to SP and/or LD. Recognizing these three, at least, phenomenological unfolding pathways toward uncanny states of consciousness may be extremely helpful when deciding which techniques to apply, or when to apply them. To be clear, these are *naturally occurring sequences* that are reported by many SP/LD experiencers regardless of how accomplished they are with other control techniques. But good shamanic timing goes a long way toward empowering the dreamer and controlling these dreams even further, so their unfolding must be known and understood.

Sequences One and Two are the most common uncanny dream unfoldings, but Sequence Three also occurs spontaneously, sometimes even before the dreamer ever recognizes his SP dreaming condition or has the anticipatory symptoms. In fact, my numbering of these sequences as 1, 2, or 3 should not be taken to represent a ranking, or any other developmental phenomenon that I am aware of. The me-shaman says, "They just happen, use them as a practical guide," whereas the scientist-shaman admits, "I have no explanation at this point about their significance." There might not be a *discursive logic* to lucid dreaming. If there is a type of "logic" it adheres to a mythological plan, but these phenomenological sequences may turn out to have more prosaic environmental or physiological underpinnings. For all three, the 'lucidness' of SP also varies from a vague and distant sensation of immobility to an intensely self-conscious experience and extreme panic. This extreme version, I guess, might feel as though one had been shot with curare: a frozen body in full consciousness.

Sequence 1

I call Sequence One the "classical" unfolding of SP-to-LD because, at least in hindsight, it is the most frequent and represents the accumulation of years of observations made. Its simplified sequence is as follows:

a) **Heaviness:** A few hours prior to bedtime
b) **'Electricity', buzzing, booming:** Within two hours prior

to bedtime; while falling asleep; and while transitioning into 'c'

c) **Sleep paralysis** proper
d) **Hallucinations**: OBEs, FOPs, incubus or on to Lucid Dreaming

Sequence 2

Sequence Two is the most annoying or terrifying, depending on your perspective, unfolding and it is characterized by a circular looping that follows this general pattern:

a) **Heaviness**: A few hours prior to bedtime
b) **'Electricity', buzzing, booming**: Within two hours prior to bedtime; while falling asleep; and while transitioning into 'c'
c) **Sleep paralysis** proper
d) **Wake UP**: OBEs, FOPs, incubus or on to Lucid Dreaming
e) **Repeats** at least two to five times decreasing until subject is to tired and falls asleep or too terrified and stays awake for the reminder of the night.

Sequence 3

Sequence Three is a rare event, indeed the "classical" unfolding of SP-to-LD because, at least in hindsight, it is the most frequent and represents the accumulation of years of observations made. Its simplified sequence is as follows:

a) **Awake**
b) **Hypnogogic hallucination as vision:** As hyper-reality of ordinary consciousness, as LD, or as OBE.
c) **Wake Up**, or continue on to LD or OBE

Although these three are the most common examples of unfolding, combinations of each are also experienced and reported. For example, the first sequence can end in a "common dream" night or even a dreamless night. Obviously what may be more important are the events that could be used as cuing proper in anticipation of creative dreaming: the sensations and conditions that led up to SP.

I did not include in this section what can be called *a fourth sequence of unfolding* because it does not occur naturally. I mentioned this sequenced earlier when I was describing the uses of mediation for the purposes of managing SP. At the end of that section I said that while using meditation prior to going to sleep, and in the absence of SP pre-dormittal symptoms (being tired, buzzing, "electricity" or body ripples), it so happens that the "shamanic" dreamer can land right into the tunnel, and experience spinning and flying sensations right away without the paralysis. When this happens at one's command, it feels as natural and mundane as riding a bicycle. In that case this voluntary sequence can be thought of as a volitional version of Sequence Three.

Epilogue to this Chapter

I have referred elsewhere in this book to the instructions in this chapter as *prescriptions* toward a healthier approach to an uncanny phenomenon. This is a bit presumptuous of me because, at best, these suggestions come mostly from my own shamanic journey; they are my own 'conjuring' and 'incantations'. It is true that others have corroborated their usefulness or have contributed an overlap of experience. But ultimately, they are *doings* earned from my subjective encounters with the uncanny, and as such, they may not alleviate the puzzlement, frustration, even suffering of other uncanny dreamers. If these suggestions do not become part of your own conjuring and empirical testing, then at least, the meditation and self hypnosis techniques outlined earlier can provide some measure of tranquility and discipline in your lives. Today we are lucky in that we can navigate through a different sort of virtual space and seek and find answers from other dreamers at the click of a "mouse." (Itself a modern totemic allusion in that mice are small enough to be able to explore through the labyrinths of knowledge.) The Internet is an oracle or a place for communicating with other shamans. We learn from one another and that is always a good thing.

On the other hand, I am very confident that while *stalking the uncanny* as a shaman-scientist the unfolding sequences of SP with LD traced earlier will be a common experience to most SP/LD dreamers. As a psychologist who believes in both a shared or communal genetic mental disposition and in unique developmental settings, I am willing to bet that many elements of the so-called-by-me shamanic journey will be the same for everyone who shares the SP syndrome. This is an important assumption, not only because it is based on the convergence of experiential data provided by the data I have received, but because at one time or another the uncanny dreamer might seek the help of a professional mental health shaman. We will benefit from his/her counsel if this counselor-as-shaman already possesses a map of the journeys we are taking. Even though this book is not based exclusively on a singular case study, case studies in medicine have proven to be useful in the initial charting of diagnosis, as templates for comparison when some 'ailment' is not known or defined. The anxiety generated by the encounters with the uncanny need to be addressed at some point, regardless.

To end on a clinical note then, the psychiatrist or psychologist treating a chronic ISP case ought to at least consider guiding the most willing and able patients into the three techniques described earlier (*SPS*), pre-dormittal self-hypnosis or other-mediated-hypnosis, and meditation-concentration techniques) with the confidence that, if successful, their patients will gain in confidence and self-esteem. *Semiotically speaking* **SPS** *is a dual sign since it can potentially convey two disparate signals: 'anxiety and fear' or 'it is now time to float about and enjoy a remarkable otherworldly dreamscape.'* Additionally, and more importantly from the experiential perspective of this author, the creative possibilities that await these subjects is more than a simple consolation for having been born with a predisposition for *bound lucidity*. It is, verily, the freedom and control to explore a noetic space to which few individuals have a natural access. As a chronic sufferer of ISP, I, and many other SP experiencers, choose to 'float about and enjoy the ride'.

Conclusion

"The earlier culture will become a heap of rubble and finally a heap of ashes, but spirits will hover over the ashes."

Wittgenstein, *Culture and Value*

The Semiotics of SP

The revolving door of everyday experience while awake, thinking that one is awake, dreaming that one is awake, and of recalling mundane dream material, with respect to the meaning transported between all four levels and their significance for person and culture, becomes a matter of semiotic interest. If semiotics is interested in deciphering the way in which these dream signs are generated, broadcast, and finally interpreted by individuals and culture, then the SP phenomena becomes a special case for this field of inquiry[67] with the added bonus that semiotics may be the only field umbrella and serious enterprise that is capable of encompassing the biology, psychology, geophysics, poetics, mythology, and cultural implications of the phenomena.

The complexity of the interaction between these levels of meaning and signification is what anthropologist and semiotician Lévi-Strauss means by *bricolage*. Lévi-Strauss co-opts the word *bricolage* from a more mundane meaning that suggests an incongruous mix that seems to hold together. By using this word Lévi-Strauss wants to convey how it is that myths might be constructed. For him (Lévi-Strauss, 1962) myths are essentially maps that assist a believer or user to use their symbols and metaphors in order to resolve or to address an experiential contradiction or conflict (always developed in the tale-myth itself). But these symbols and metaphors must come from somewhere. Lévi-Strauss thinks of the obvious— that myths are built from the kaleidoscopic multiplicity of social and environmental facts or activities. Others have advanced the idea that dreams are also a *bricolage* (Kracke, 1987). The difference between the mythic and dream compositions of reality is that the myth is more static than the *bricolage* of the dream. The bricolage of the dream, especially when it is aided by the dreamer's willful control of the dreamscape, ceases to be simply another social item, but a transcendental, tool often times risking facile social interpretations. In traditional cultures where taboos are respected and the norms are tight and inflexible, the bricolage of the controlled, self-aware dream may be one of the few methods of challenging myths that cease to guide with wisdom precisely because dreaming is itself, if not a shamanic journey, an ancestral form of communication. This is Lévi-Strauss' *mythical thought.*

Both myths and dreams contain creatively and synthetically formulated "truths" that have the potential of guiding the development of self. Joseph Campbell said, "The myth is the public dream and the dream is the private myth." In that sense both myth and dreaming need and feed off each other. *So there are enduring and universal existential realities apprehended by a personal and basic human psychobiology that can become heuristics or archetypal truths. It is certain that the personal and private dream machine reflects (acknowledges) these archetypal truths. But it is also the case that it has the capacity to invent new ones or provide new images for old ones. In this sense "Big Dreaming" is an awesome enterprise and responsibility, on equal footing with any creative human enterprise because it uses the individual-as-a-dreamer as a new and contemporary interpretant of old mythology to infuse into old social patterns new rituals, signs, symbols and behavioral repertoires.* Logically, this process of mythical renewal also means that sometimes the private dream world is in conflict with the public myth, a situation that Mythologist Joseph Campbell thinks can lead to trouble: neurosis. Campbell writes that individuals confronting this neurosis have been visionaries, leaders and heroes. In a passage that could be a summary for this book—for the creative potentials for SP and LD that I have been arguing for, including the obstacles that need to be overcome—he further describes the resolution of this neurosis as follows:

"They've [visionaries, leaders and heroes] moved out of the society that would have protected them, and into the dark forest, into the world of fire, of original experience. Original experience has not been interpreted for you, and so you've got to work out your life yourself. Either you can take it or you can't. You don't have to go far off the interpreted path to find yourself in very difficult situations. The courage to face the trials and to bring a whole new body of possibilities into the field of interpreted experience for other people to experience-that is the hero's deed."

At yet another level, the biological, humans are animals, designated by species, family and genus. We are primates, and our uncanny dreaming and dreaming states served in the adaptations of many species before us. If SP, LD, or a rich dreaming life are phenomena still manifesting themselves in our experiential makeup then it is because they were useful adaptations. Then understanding their genesis and potential for problem solving and personal unfolding becomes a practical and even necessary enterprise. But always, it seems to me, these dream experiences are the precursors of what Lévi-Strauss calls the mythical. In this primal and important sense, people who are lucky enough to experience them as everyday or continuing realities are privy to truly archaic knowledge modes that deserve to be understood even more so because of their primacy and their enduring status in addition to any tools they provide for problem solving and personal growth. *Mythical thought* is the observation of "a sensible world in sensible terms."

As the opening quote by Wittgenstein suggests, the semiosis of SP as a study includes the exploration of the pernicious quality and intensity of the experience, a common psychobiological cause, and its enduring manifestation: lifetime and historical, psychological effects. That is, *even after the material elements of cultures cease, there remains a psychobiology of SP as hovering spirits, that make their reappearance in another culture, in another time, described using vernacular terminology. The new and vernacular terminology and experiences can be adopted into new myths or can modify the old ones. Thus, the bricolage of myth is reconstituted anew.*

Moreover, when aspects of dreaming become hyperconscious through SP or LD, then, semiotically speaking, convoluted, grasping-at-straws psychoanalysis[68] has less to contribute to our study because paralysis is paralysis is paralysis, manifested and felt, without hidden meanings. "I am frozen, I cannot move or wake up," internally screams the SP sufferer. *This is not an unconsciously generated hysterics but a bodily humor gone tainted.* Now I must interpret for myself or with the help of poetry, myth and culture what being frozen means *for me.* Furthermore, it helps the dreamer if others have made a similar journey and have practical advice to dispense. This is a semiotic process that owes some debt to psychoanalysis, as long as psychoanalysis or other clinical attempts are not second-guessing SP as anything less than a bodily reality. But as we will see later the founders of psychoanalysis were well grounded in mythology and in the study of its manifestation within.

As we have seen in previous chapters, the sign "I am frozen" cannot be communicated, or is only partially communicated to someone else. The sign, "I am frozen," has a double meaning to the experiencer: it could mean I am hopeless, alone, and afraid; or I think it is time to play, to fly, to begin lucid dreaming. Only through experience, tutelage, and self-discovery can this sign "I am frozen" become anything else than "trouble ahead, in the dark."

With rare exceptions, the phenomenology of SP is at a rich and complex semiotic journey and cross roads, because there exists the potential for a very personal and subjective interpretation of the experience, and at the same time, there is a potential resolution to the meaning of being paralyzed given what "others" say it is about.

To all this one must accept the likelihood that Freud is basically correct when he repeatedly makes the argument that dreams have an energy charge that belongs more to the infantile than to the rational or adult basically because the infantile registered its first universe, for months and years at a time, enveloped in purely perceptual and sensorial truths. By this we should not infer that this infantile mode is less precise at conveying truths, or remembering trauma, or that it has no role to play in adult life and in the development of self.

To conveniently deny this early and rich existence and assume that it plays no part in dreaming life—an experience inundated with pure sensation, perceptions, and undifferentiated scenes that are hard to discern and control—is at least bad science. Thus, leaving this developmental aspect out of the SP-dream *bricolage* makes it more difficult to explain the phenomenology of the dream content as being expressed in strong emotions, in visual or sensorial tones, and always stuck in the present.

The SP and LD experiencers are once again in a unique position of experiential advantage and potential psychological growth because they can continue to develop in dream states. *Using Freud's model again, these dream shamans can bring to submission the fuzzy and busy infantile aspect of the average dream, forge at will, or by technique, and daily practice into another consciousness state where self-awareness has an extended opportunity to evolve with new experiences.* If one is troubled by the simplistic, imperfect, and unfortunate man-in-the-street rendition of Freud's idea of the infantile in the dream I urge you to consider an alternative interpretation. My interpretation, a thought experiment, asks that you pretend to be a big cat, monkey, or whatever animal you identify with (it has to be a mammal), and imagine what its dreams would be like. I imagine that its dreams would be about its strong limbic system reactions to its existence for sure, joys and fears, all these played out in an eternal tense: the present. Its ideas would be also rooted in the perceptual or the sensorial rather than on higher order, rational thought processes. Its motoric agility, real, remembered or desired, may take the form of a sort of flying, in flight or fight or chase. I am not saying that human dreaming, shamanic or not, cannot be more than these experiences, but I am saying that Freud, by looking at the "infantile" as a significant source of dreaming, has connected all animal minds to our animal mind and made it possible to think about the origins of our human totemic experiences. By sharing these evolutionary dreaming predispositions the shamanic is simply a natural and logical expression of that collective. I will try to develop this point further in the next section.

Freudian and Jungian Bricolage

Freud, like a wise and savvy old shaman, ends *The Interpretation of Dreams* with what is, in my opinion, the best chapter in that immense book. He saves his best trick for the end. The long and complex chapter, "The Psychology of the Dream Process[69]," contains a revolutionary section (B) simply entitled "Regression"[70]. But his meaning of the word regression in this section is not what it is usually and first thought of, as in a regression to infantile or juvenile behavioral or cognitive states. He means by this term a hypothetical neuronal mechanism of regressing to perceptual-sensorial states from conscious states involving motor volition and control during dreaming. The reverse order of this neuronal process is engaged while we are awake. At the risk of oversimplifying a 'must read' by anyone who thinks Freud is outdated and has little to contribute to psychobiology and cognition, he proposes, ahead of his time, a neurocognitive model that attempts to sketch a series of perceptual, memory and motoric systems arranged in a precise and logical sequence. These arrangements of systems representing the psyche are introduced as a theory of dreams that Freud thinks may account for empirically observable facts. For example, the flow of information to and from the ends of this processing of information (one end being the capturing of physical stimuli by sensorial mechanism the other being consciousness itself) determines whether we are dreaming, hallucinating or engaged in ordinary reality. In the same model, he not only provides reasons why this cognitive regression flow terminates during dreaming, in the exploration of images and old memories or the visual images of older memories, but argues convincingly why this is an "infantile"[71] mode.

Simply put, Freud reaches the conclusion that thoughts are transformed into visual images when we dream. Furthermore, in an important declaration he says, "... we may describe the dream as the substitute for the infantile scene modified by transference to recent material. The infantile scene cannot enforce its own revival, and must therefore be satisfied to return as a dream." The process of transference is important here for Freud as well because it is the bridge that will connect and recombine into a new bricolage two seemingly unrelated events that share common elements. Transference is a semiotic process of association of meaning.

Thus, in a real semiotic sense he is providing a hypothesis

and a neurocognitive model that might explain the so-called alien abduction phenomena in the context of experiencing SP. If I interpret his model correctly, the sign "paralysis" acts as an important and loud signal in contrast to the expected motoric output, mobility itself, and sends the dreamer into an immediate matching recollection of a similar event in the past. *The visual memories that are reformulated are not of past and real encounters with gray-green aliens from another planet, but of the first afterbirth encounter with perceptually distorted human beings.* If a sensitive individual had experienced his/her birth trauma and remembers more details than the average person and also experiences SP, then Freud's model predicts that the outcome will be a seek-and-match visual memory that seems to explain the present situation, sleep paralysis. But as he argued earlier, this special type of dreamer also has the capacity to seek other dreamscapes and to control any other image while in consciousness. From adding new cultural components and suggestions to ignoring these inputs and creating a new dream experience, the special and uncanny dreamer is poised to revisit alien visitation stories at the prompting of the SP signal or to journey deeper into the unconscious.

Freud may have overreached with other psychological ideas, but he seems to identify important universals in dreaming that, if not related to a truly ancestral source, point to primitive and animal-like cerebral processes we may share with at least all mammals. If so, then it makes sense that dreams are more akin to traditional shamanic experiences and lore because they demand from the dreamer a different psychological attitude that includes and results in totemism, in the expression of universals in totemic form. This pre-historical and historical process, in twists and turns that may not be recognizable to the modern or untrained eye, is the *archetypal psychohistory* discovered by Jung's insight into psychology and mythology, or as Edward F. Edinger puts it, "the self-manifestation of the archetypes of the collective unconscious as they emerge and develop in time and space through the actions and fantasies of humanity."

This process of *archetypal psychohistory* is, in my opinion, multiplied many times over, magnified, incremented, intensified, accelerated, made concrete, brought forth, and encapsulated in the person who experiences SP and LD. Shamanism is then the flesh-and-bones intimate process of identification, through totemism, with universals and SP/LD its non-pharmaceutical vehicle.

If totemic, the symbols and language signs endure, clamoring, as a connection to the animal within by representing its aspects through mythological pantheons that span human experience. From these symbols, I choose two—one from the west and one from the east—to advertise the potential for SP and LD to facilitate or to make these discoveries possible.

Jung and Campbell and many others have analyzed the examples that follow with better credentials and erudition than I, rooting them in classical literature and the workings of the psyche. But as a mere neophyte on this path, I choose them, today, because they succinctly describe MY experiences. The example from the west is Aion, the winged torso of a man with the head of a lion, encircled by a serpent, and resting on an egg (the myth of Phanes will work as well). The symbolism for SP/LD, for me, is of the struggle of the psyche of the shaman emanating from a primordial and ineffable source (egg) to reach the heavens and elucidation (flying, lucid dreaming), while constrained by the grip of the serpent (snake). The physical body is thus constrained but other aspects of the entire psyche and are not are allowed to pursue knowledge. The head of the lion represents the courage needed to venture into these realms and knowledge. In short, and as Campbell points out, the existential struggle of reaching maturity and passing through developmental stages is that of a conflict between an eagle that must soar and the serpent that tries to hold it down. Once again, in my interpretation the eagle stands for LD and the serpent for SP. A resolution of this conflict, Campbell says, is that of a synthesis and the meaning of transcendence: a winged dragon expressing both aspects of unfolding and being. Thus the dragon could represent the mastery of the shaman.

My second example comes, once again, from Jung and Campbell. The Eastern image related in the Upanishads illustrates Vishnu as a sleeping god, who every now and then gives birth to the (a) universe, a lotus that grows and blossoms out of its navel. Brahman, the creator, sits on the blossom and then, "Brahman opens his eyes, and a world comes into being." (Campbell, 1988.) This second and possible symbol for SP and LD is equally powerful for ME, more so because the deities are both dreaming and from their dreaming the stuff of the universe and all possibility emerge. When Vishnu pleases, according to an incomprehensible will or plan, the lotus dies and the possibility of Brahman and creation with it. The photograph I am now looking at comes from Jung's book, Symbols of Transformation, and is part of a relief from Vijayanagar, India. In this image, too, Vishnu rests on a multi-headed cobra whose heads are raised above Vishnu's as if in a gesture of protection and grounding

As in the image of Aion, the symbolism for me is almost a mnemonic to remind us (ME) that transcendence begins with a grounding, in our presentation forced by the spontaneous SP experience, culminating in an act of creation, illumination, and expansion—what follows during and after the LD experiences.

Parting Thoughts: ". . . spirits will hover over the ashes."

Echoing our earlier claims about the ancestral and even phylogenetic primacy of the SP and LD experiences, Freud speculates that, "Behind this childhood of the individual we are then promised an insight into the phylogenetic childhood, into the evolution of the human race, of which the development of the individual is only an abridged repetition influenced by the fortuitous circumstances of life." A few lines later in this passage Freud goes on to quote Friedrich Nietzsche as confirming his insight. In the words of Nietzsche, "there persists a primordial part of humanity which we can no longer reach by a direct path." The path Freud hopes Nietzsche is referring to is dreaming life as a bridge connecting us to a primordial ecological unconscious. Intrigued by Freud's need to quote Nietzsche while making his claim I researched Nietzsche and found the following passage in All-Too-Human:

"In the ages of the rude beginnings of culture, man believed that he was discovering a second real world in dream, and here is the origin of metaphysics. Without dream, mankind would never have had occasion to invent such a division of the world. The parting of soul and body goes also with this way of interpreting dream; likewise, the idea of a soul's apparitional body: whence, all belief in ghosts, and apparently, too, in gods."

Additionally, while in putting a plug for psychoanalysis itself, Freud declares, "It would seem that dreams and neuroses have preserved for us more of the psychical antiquities than we suspected; so that psychoanalysis may claim a high rank among those sciences which endeavored to reconstruct the oldest and darkest phases of the beginnings of mankind." As we saw before, this endeavor is Jung's *archetypal psychohistory* analysis that inspects the dream material and content, and analyzes its relation to the material and content of established myths.

I suppose I am arguing from authority here only because I cannot make any of you dream my dreams nor live my myths. If you did dream in the context of bound lucidity, liberated by lucid dreaming flight and while using the techniques described in this book or those described by others, then their embrace would feel ancient indeed. If you were to dream

these dreams—my uncanny, terrible, and wonderful dreams—
the journey toward transcendence I referred to in Chapter
Four, as one of the shamanic, empirical principles, might, with
time, present and introduce the following symbols and deeds
as signposts along a road of transformation also in you:

1) *Nature-at-large or the natural will gain in prominence and
   importance until one becomes ecologically in tune or can no
   longer accept the artificial.* By artificial I mean a journey
   away from the origin of the myth or a forgetting that results
   in embracing shallow and superficial undertakings.
   Nature's call finally overrides social pantomime.

2) *The jaguar (animus) chases a deer (anima), they dance around
   and around each other until they become incorporated into a
   circle signifying the need for transcendence as unification and
   individuation.* The opposites are integrated or ambiguity
   is accepted. Totemic wisdom is accepted as part of the
   natural order.

3) *Multicolor lines emanating from every living thing rise
   above the plains and waters and are entangled into oneness:
   they represent all life.* More importantly, the intertwining
   of these lifelines represents the unity of all life into a
   grander ecological bricolage. Nature's pain becomes
   one's pain, her exhibitions is also our knowledge.

4) *Absolute silence will overcome you and while being engulfed
   in the disappearance of all forms, you still find a
   "something" that stands for a better instance of yourself:
   an original form.* Through this silence and subsequent
   rebirth one discovers the falsity of culture as an engine
   for layering in many false personas. I am the I.

5) *The eyes of a cougar will meet yours, he will test you, chase
   you, even bite you. Next time around when you encounter
   him, he will invite you to ride on his back and will show
   you worlds beyond imagination.* The totemic relation

engenders both respect for other life forms and a willingness to accept their existences as instruction that can be incorporated in the human act of survival. A human animal recognizes its ancestry.

6) *Older dream-uncanny folks, men or women, will come and teach you with patience, usually, pragmatic maneuvers that facilitate further control in the dream world.* These entities can be archetypical and knowable or brand new manifestations of our own psychical experience or present need. Either way they are poised to remind, cajole, instruct, admonish, and always guide when no one else can. The 'stranger' helps.

With this knowledge and more, one is better disposed and able to get up in the morning and face a world that "seems" mundane, chaotic or senseless, and *see* in it instead grandiose historical or existential scales: rhythms, cycles, the inevitability and stupidity of mortality, the folly of the superficial and over prescribed.

Throughout this book, the science of SP and LD was revisited, the personal was related, the stories and journeys of others included, the pragmatic approaches presented, the so-called supernatural was, hopefully, demystified.

But in this conclusion, I can find no more satisfying outcome or compromise than the final realization and continued publicizing that Freud, Jung and so many others have proposed: *the gaining of courage for pursuing these psychic transformations as part of a grander **aesthetic semiotic process**. We can refer to this becoming as one of reacquiring an **ecological consciousness** with the totality of our being that also includes the activities of all other beings, virtual or natural.* This is exercising our mythical thinking abilities.

To all those efforts, I have humbly added another consideration, namely, that the dual experiences of SP and

LD could be quick and natural shortcuts to achieve these transformations, and by implication, that the dysfunctions that originate in SP and LD should not be treated, but reinforced, channeled, and made into positive "sorcery."

Another contribution was the connection, tenuous at this point I must admit, that geomagnetic forces have also played a part in our archetypical history. More specifically, that these forces are triggers of the SP experience and can anticipate its neurology. If this puzzle piece is found to be valid or real, it assists, expands and brings the old shamanic knowledge to include a scientifically testable hypothesis about an intimate dialectic between the planetary and the cosmos and the personal or psychobiological. Thus scientific inquiry and mythical thinking are conjoined.

Not that the old shamans needed geoscience or neuropsychology to confirm the intimations that they always knew and talked about. But as a scientist and a mythical dreamer, my aesthetic sense is that much more aggrandized. That is, I expand my own scientific and personal experiences into a *grander aesthetic semiotic process*.

Bound lucidity, Aion or Vishnu, is a trans-cultural phenomenon always pointing in the direction of "big" images and "big" themes. Some of you may still argue, "it may only feel as though your dreams belonged to some ancient realm, but it is just your imagination." Then permit me to say that these dreams are at least inspiring, and allow me to leave you with this poem for your troubles, and simply call my dreams "poems":

The shaman of Oblieng[72]

Sleep of day
Sleep of tender
Sleep of me-wolves
Who surrender

> to fragments of unimaginable fright.

Sleep of winded leaves
Sleep of Berserkers drinking
With the me-sages
Drinking moon milk

           so that others go mad.

Sleep of tossing
Sleep of flying
Sleep of disappearance
From this world

           in the fangs of the shaman of
           Oblieng.

Sleep of instinct
Sleep without rules
Sleep otherworldly
Sleep of death

           sleep of being awake inside the
           chambers of one's heart.

Sleep feline
Sleep ancient
Sleep temple
Sleep jade

           like the Olmecs wore jade with
           jaguar faces.

Sleep of new moon
When the owls are silent
When the wind implodes
When the soil goes insane

           when the trees carve themselves
           a grave in my chest.

Sleep of all sleepers
All whispering at the same time
The nonsense of yesteryears
Prisoners of their own beds.
Sleep of frozen waters
Sleep of walking alone

In the steppes
With the Olmecs
In Oblieng
With fox-fur sandals
Drinking moon milk
Devouring owls
Being a corpse
Enduring this short death.
Sleep not night
But Fly

EPILOGUE

Questions and Hypotheses in Need of Answers and Some Tentative Proposals

"There is nothing so practical as a good theory."

-Kurt Lewin

'The drunken man looked for his lost wallet underneath the street lamp because the light was better there."

-Paraphrased from Abraham Kaplan

Questions About LD, Flying, Sex, and Everything Else

I call this last section an epilogue because it is really another door or many doors opening simultaneously to further scientific work and inquiry. The scientist and the shaman in me need additional answers to questions that I have been asked by others or have posited on my own. I am not going to elaborate on the first set of questions, Section A, too much; instead, I invite the interested reader, the graduate student, or the co-researcher to ponder them as anti-koans in need of clarification. I do elaborate on an additional set of questions in the next section, Section B, partly because these are ongoing in my research and I would like to pursue some of them. By asking them here, I am giving you a head start and

189

insight into my own curiosity and future endeavors, I would also welcome anyone else to pursue these questions as well. Let me know what you find out. The last section of this epilogue, Section C, is both a real and a hypothetical dialogue between a colleague and myself as a way of addressing questions the reader may have asked throughout this book.

Section A: I Would Like to Explore the Following

1) Why is it that "flying" is a universal experience in LD? Humans don't fly; we walk, run or crawl, so why would "flying" be so intensely our experience?[73]

2) In what way is physiological (autonomic) sexual arousal during REM sleep related or causal to the sensation of flying?

3) Specifically, are there neuronal systems that, during sexual arousal in REM sleep and because of the atonic condition of REM, are expressed as a different motor output: flying?

4) Specifically, are there neuronal systems that are already engaged during sexual arousal, copulation, and the experience of an orgasm while awake that give rise to sensory or motor activations that mimic the feeling of flying? Why should there be a connection?

5) Specifically, does the wealth of traditional (romantic non-fiction and fictional) lore and literature about sexuality, copulation and orgasm, metaphorically employ flying as a byproduct of pleasurable acts? If so, why, once again, would "flying" be connected with the romantic sexual experience?

6) Is "flying" a necessary cognitive construct, a particular form of mobility that is engaged when the body is paralyzed during REM sleep?

7) Is "flying" a necessary cognitive construct, a particular form of mobility that is engaged when the body is

paralyzed during REM sleep AND we lay prone on a surface?

8) Are some of the acoustic perceptions reported in SP magnifications of bodily functions (high-pitched noises in the ear, breathing, pulse, heart beat, stomach growls, etc.)?

9) Is the sensation of going through tunnels correlated with being under covers, sheets, sleeping bags, etc.[74]?

10) Connected with any of the above specific questions and thinking back to Freud's explanation that vivid dreams can be *Hyper-amnesic Dreams* and infantile sensations and visual impressions that survive strongly in our respective psychologies, then is the experience of flying, or of flying and autonomic sexual arousal during REM sleep, the experience of going through tunnels, spinning, etc., connected as a huge semiotic code to the birthing experience?

Section B: Further Work: Clinical, Occupational, Psychobiological, Neurological and Interdisciplinary (Geomagnetic, Folkloric, Historical)

More theoretical and empirical work needs to take place with respect to the following:

1) The incidence of SP in SP-prone individuals who start taking Zoloft, Prozac, or any other antidepressant before and after they took these pharmaceuticals.

2) Put a number on the incidence of SP among long-haul truck drivers, transcontinental airplane crews, or any other job-related situation that demands that normal sleep be significantly altered: postponed, lost and/or distorted.

3) Identification of people who claim to have birth memories independently from reporting so-called

alien abduction phenomena or even SP. Compare their recollections to the narratives of the so-called alien abduction phenomena.

4) Multiple disciplines (medicine, psychobiology, clinical psychology, etc.) and further efforts need to take a closer look at the psychobiology, neurology, psychology, and the entire dreaming ecology of the so-called alien abductee. Specifically, SP if identified with this experience, needs to be explained in the context of *Hyperamnesic Dreams,* infantile sensations, and visual impressions that might have survived strongly in their respective psychologies.

5) Professionally appropriate and self-empowering uses of hypnotherapy are to be sought and continued in order to cope with SP and to elucidate its ecology. These efforts include using hypnotherapy as a first step in self-hypnosis training, for creating *anchoring techniques* (see Chapter Five), and for helping in visualization and relaxation with the aim of reducing stress or facilitating movement from SP into LD (also in Chapter Five). The reports, successes and failures, resulting from using hypnotherapy in this way may provide much needed information about other situations in which SP occurs, may help gather demographics data, or may supply any missing data not presently available.

6) Related to undertaking efforts One through Five, hypnotherapy needs to be revisited as a clinical tool and even suspected as a poor medium for obtaining objective information about SP. Specifically, the work of practitioners who, without scientific, psychiatric and clinical training, or with no interest in testing and discarding improbable hypotheses, needs to be critiqued and further inspected. This is not a trivial undertaking given the fact that the first encounter

(pun intended) with the hypnotherapist about the SP experience for many sufferers may be overhearing a popular portrayal of small sized beings with nefarious intentions. In order to curtail the impact of these popular effects we professionals must repeat the following, scientifically/clinically sensible mantras:

6i)   We are dealing with a multifaceted and highly dynamic psychological experience.

6ii) This already biased experience is rooted in the complex and shifting realities of the crossroads of consciousness during transitions between awake, semi-awake, REM, REM and SP, REM and SP and LD, and hypnogogic hallucinations.

6iii) The incidence of SP already comes with a building history of psychological and cultural adaptation, personal trauma, and perhaps other dysfunctions.

6iv) Popular practitioners, with motives other than to empower individuals and dreamers or test falsifiable theories and hypotheses, may endanger rather than help a client with a potentially understandable and manageable condition and life experience. These practitioners and their dubious methods and unknown motivations need to be openly criticized as frequently as possible. Their methods and interpretations are of no service to the cause of seeking or maintaining psychological well being.

6v)   The long-term and creative possibilities of SP and LD need to be kept in mind as a continued source of psychological unfolding and becoming.

6vi) The long-term and creative possibilities of SP and LD need to be naturally folded or, knitted tightly into an already present set of principles that have been termed "shamanic" or "New Age" but nevertheless express the more beneficial and historically enduring wisdom of past dream-uncanny experiencers.

7) Multiple, additional, and convergent tests and other empirical connections, including those of an experimental, narrative, anecdotal, or historical-archival nature, need to be conducted in order to continue to test the hypothesis that the incidence of reporting SP and LD increases or decreases during abrupt changes in the geomagnetic field

8) Knowing and /or assuming that: a) the circumpolar and Tioga-tundra regions and their traditional inhabitants (or historically recent but permanent residents) such as the Inuit and Simi are exposed to more intense and abrupt geomagnetic conditions, electromagnetic, and atmospherics conditions that people of other regions do not encounter; and b) that the same circumpolar and Tioga-tundra inhabitants go through extreme changes in daylight conditions that could create REM-rebound conditions or extended darkness and sleep patterns:

8i)   Do these populations report a higher incidence of SP and LD?

8ii) If 8i is true, do these populations' folklore reflect this increased incidence?

8iii) If 8i or 8ii are true, are the shamanic lore and practices particularly sensitive to these changes?

9) More information needs to be gathered that tests the "ring of fire" hypothesis of a greater incidence of SP and its folklore occurring in the geomagnetically active Pacific regions.

10) The incidence of SP in all of these SP-prone populations and groups needs to be compared to the incidence of the sleep disorder in other geomagnetic

and/or photo circadian stable regions (the tropics for example).

11) Some hallucinogenic substances such as Mandrake, Datura, the cactus San Pedro, and others have been reported to produce sensations of flying or are taken in order to embark on a sorcerous/shamanic journey. Are cerebral systems (such as the motor and sensory cortices or vestibular systems) particularly affected by the ingestion of these substances? If so, are the same neuronal systems engaged during SP, LD and LD with flying?

12) A collection of SP narratives needs to be gathered, when SP is suspected, from the very young, in an unbiased way, trying to capture the evolution of the experience from a personal and uncontaminated source to its relation to an existing cultural milieu.

13) There might be an additional common psychological "protection" against SP and so-called alien abduction experiences, *a self-correcting and developmental mechanism based on increased maturity and dealing with life in general.* It is interesting to me that even in the so-called alien abduction scenario, long-term abductees' narratives are later transformed into more benign and even uplifting experiences that include environmental, transformational, mystical, or practical narrative themes. This developmental coping pattern is discussed in the alien abduction literature. Because this presumed developmental and coping maturity with the uncanny transcends the SP, shamanic, and so-called alien abduction experiences, then the content reflected by this evolution becomes less important and this lifespan cognitive-affective process can be explained (may have already been explained) by psychological theory.

14) Related to number eight, given that Earth's geomagnetic field, according to accumulating data of the past one

hundred years, is waning, in some regions of the planet more significantly than in others (noticeably in the southern hemisphere, the so-called South Atlantic Anomaly)[75], then are the inhabitants of these geomagnetically changing regions reporting the prevalence of SP differently; is the prevalence of SP more than should be expected? (All the geomagnetic hypotheses listed here and in my other reports are/can be further testing of Persinger's geopsychological and geopsychopathological theses, 1987. For example, my 'ring of fire' hypothesis is a logical test of his proposals.)

Section C: Final Questions, Final Answers

During a presentation of my ecopsychological ideas, a researcher, author and colleague of mine whom I respect asked me a question that I will now repeat and adapt to the SP situation. After several attempts at an acceptable answer I broke down his complex and important question into its components, resulting in these questions:

1) What do we gain as modern people in revisiting, reliving or reverting back to natural or ancestral modes of being and psychologically relating?

2) Can our psychological systems, accustomed to new techno-ecologies, even remember how to relate to these ancestral modes?

3) Are ancestral humans, or humans living naturally today, happier and more fulfilled than you and I, civilized scientists, are?

4) How can we even test a hypothetical improved condition of reverting back to an ancestral mode of psychological being when we subjectively flow into the new being state? (Anthropologists and their critics speak of this condition as one of being subjectively

embedded in a culture to such a degree that the
possibility for comparison is not even possible.)

5) Isn't psychological well-being or dysfunction culturally
relative? By that principle, are our western cures
appropriate for our western maladies?

In one way or another I believe I have already attempted to
address some of my colleague's concerns or versions of the
questions posited above with respect to the writings in this entire
book. But as a way of recapitulating and summarizing lengthier
passages here are the same questions and some answers:

1) What does a person who suffers from SP and does not
know it, but believes he/she has been abducted by
aliens (thanks to the efforts of dubious and biased
hypnotherapy), gain by becoming a modern "sorcerer"
or "shaman"? Isn't this really leaving one delusion to
embrace another; going from the frying pan into the
fire?

Answer: In my mind, there isn't a terminus, an "arriving at"
existential questions/answers. That is, self-actualization
is a never-ending process. Thus, by taking on a pro-
active, volitional and disciplined way, by embracing *the
archetype of the shaman* on the way to testing universal
psychological truths, we are empowering individuals who
might be either ignorant, confused, or preoccupied for
the wrong reasons. It is certainly a bonus if along the
way they also learn mediation, self-hypnosis and find,
as in "The Wizard of Oz," their courage.

2) Which is better; the psychological, cultural, or creative
gains that able practitioners and controllers of SP and
LD obtain despite the obstacles they have to overcome
to get there, or the quick and modern pharmaceutical
fix that allows reality to be predictable, controllable, and
stress free 24/7?

Answer: I run outdoors on country trails and have long abandoned the paved streets, the cushy tracks or indoor lanes for the unpredictable and challenging dirty, muddy, and complex tracks of nature. In the many years I have been doing this, I have noticed that my senses are sharper, that my instincts and reactions to surprising changes on this wild path have become more authentic, quicker, and more appropriate. My body and mind have conformed to the nuances and complexity of natural spaces with gains that are transferable to other aspects of my life. In contrast, I know that humanity did not evolve in predictable, controllable, and stress free environments, social or natural, 24/7.

Does not therapy that aims at returning us to health and ancient patterns need to give us these tools, or steer us in this direction? The "cushy" path is fine for some if these individuals have been forced to be so synthetic and dependent on the artificial and the external that nothing else equates with well being. But this is an aberration of ideal health.

3)   Are some of the ancient skills we referred to as "shamanic" beneficial at all? Couldn't they in fact be harmful to a western mind now decontextualized from a natural setting and prohibited by local laws to explore these realms?

Answer: Harmful? Absolutely not, given the restricted sense of what I have explored and described as shamanic: in the context of beginning to experience SP and then having to deal with this condition as a lifetime syndrome. In the context of this book, and for the purposes of controlling the SP/LD experiences, these practices are, generally speaking, beneficial and are not, generally speaking, harmful. I am cautious here because individuals vary with respect to their physical or psychological constitution and for some the shamanic path may bring additional stress and anxiety. For these individuals, then the pharmaceutical route may be the only path to health.

On the other hand, if we look at all the shamanic practices that have been passed down to us or at the ones that exist today, then the answer is also, it depends. That is, it depends on what one means by "beneficial" or "harmful". For example, taking hallucinogens in certain societies for "shamanic purposes" will get you into legal trouble. This is the case even in our hypocritical USA where locals ingest volumes of alcohol for no sane or healthy purpose whatsoever, and where Native American Religions, for example, have been allowed to pursue these agents within the context of their religion. But I have not advocated the use of these agents here. The SP/LD experiencer is naturally endowed with the mystical and needs no such help. Going back to my earlier point, and speaking about western, industrialized nations, fewer and fewer material sacred things/objects, modern-day customs, life styles, housing accommodations, or ritualized practices tie us to these ancestral ways.

We live in an age of facile thermostatic and illusory control of nature and the ancestral being is forgotten today. But biology and psychology are tied and cannot be changed superficially or so quickly. *The SP/LD experiences are not merely vestiges of a long gone era of natural adaptation, but rather are loud voices that clamor as loudly today as they always have about an intimate connection we have only forgotten about.*

4) Can we allow proficient SP and LD dreamers to claim that they are better off today having conquered their fears, and manipulating creatively a fascinating dreamscape, than the alien abductee, who sits in group sessions talking about the last abduction or anticipating in fear the next

kidnapping? Since the SP and LD evolution lands them in a uniquely subjective position, are they even entitled to make this claim?

Answer: By any reasonable, objective and aesthetic account the following have to be seen as improvements:

a) Flying is better than being frozen and helpless any day (unless you are a rock, but I can imagine that even rocks enjoy being hurled through the air from time to time).

b) Some claim that meditating and having orgasms in dreamscapes are far more intense and of higher quality than in the mortal realm; I agree. Instead of this being a social disconnecting force in waking reality the dreamscape experiences give rise to the need to explore the terrestrial versions at a higher level of proficiency, quality, intimacy, pleasure, and transformation.

c) Meditating and having orgasms in dreamscapes have to feel better than being kidnapped by aliens then strapped to a metal table and forced into strange medical-sexual practices that mostly hurt (unless you dig that sort of thing).

d) Being talked down to by the John Mackes of the world, in a boorish academic and self-assured way, is less exciting than learning to ride a magical deer into outer space and playing ethereal music that one can then reproduce and sell for profit in waking reality.

e) Staring down a hairy beast or ghost and making them look or run away, while in an OBE, is a victory that may make its way into the waking confidence of the dreamer. Likewise, being stared at by dark pit less eyes, then talked down to, then alien-handled, and shot at by all shapes and species of extraterrestrials against one's will, again and again, is bound to impact the waking confidence of the dreamer.

f) Wrestling a hairy beast or ghost down to the floor and winning, while in an OBE, is a victory that may make its way into the waking confidence of the dreamer. Likewise, being abducted, then frozen, then tele-transported, and fondled by all shapes and species of extraterrestrials against one's will, again and again, is bound to impact the waking confidence of the dreamer.

5) Isn't psychological well-being or dysfunction culturally relative? By that principle, aren't our western cures appropriate for our western maladies?

Answer: If by western remedies we mean the little blue and the bigger yellow pills that pharmaceutical companies and some modern day shamans are forcing us to ingest to make everything "disappear", then these are not cures but maladies themselves, an example of societal changes gone mad! If the modern MD—Shamans, for all practical purposes, *work for* the companies that sell the little blue and the bigger yellow pills, then they have abandoned us, and we mythical, wise, and ancient shamans should not want any part in their economy. *The only blue or yellow I want in my life is sky and water or sunsets and wild mustard flowers.*

If by culture-relative one refers to the 'surface' of psychology, ontogeny, then it is certainly the case that every human belongs to a culture. But questionable cultural practices, and the effects they have on an ideal and healthy psychobiological teleology and potential, can be criticized when they fail to support self-empowering ways and when they become an obstacle to the universal shamanic objectives: *Flying journeys to*

Lower and Upper worlds with sleep paralysis as a catalyst, seeking visions and finding an authentic form of ecstasy that expands courage and intelligence.

NOTES

Introduction

1   They are often reported while taking an afternoon nap, and specifically, while sleeping on one's back.

2   —David J. Ness, *The Terror That Comes In The Night: An Experience-centered Study of the Supernatural Assault Traditions*. Philadelphia: University of Pennsylvania press, 1982.

    —Robert C. Ness, "The Old Hag Phenomenon as Sleep Paralysis: A Biocultural Interpretation," *Culture, medicine and Psychiatry*, 2 (1978): 26-28.

3   For the first two chapters and this introduction I will use the terms "sufferer" and "experiencer" interchangeably. However, as the reader will discover this book is about transforming the more passive phenomenology of the SP as a "sufferer" into a dreamer/ empiricist who can learn to control these experiences, to a more neutral "experiencer" of the phenomenon.

4   If not abbreviated, the phrase "sleep paralysis" will be employed to refer to its normal, unconscious physiological function during REM sleep.

5   Depending on the individual dreamer, this could be up to three hours during a full, average night of sleep-7-8 hours.

6   Dr. Rodney Radtke testified on Mr. Jones's behalf in the State of North Carolina v. Stephen Clay Jones, Sr. (case No. COA99-437, April 4, 2000) after he diagnosed a REM Sleep Disorder. For other cases similar to Mr. Jones' the reader may want to read articles written by Dr. Carlos H. Schenck. Dr. Schenck is an associate professor of psychiatry, University of Minnesota Medical School, Minneapolis, Minnesota.

7   A topic of consideration in itself, a graduate student at the Depart-
     ment of Speech Communication at The Pennsylvania State Uni-
     versity, Corinne Weisgerber, has explored the issue of self-diagno-
     sis using the internet in a paper entitled, *Turning to the Internet for
     Medical Problems: The Case of the Online Sleep Paralysis Community.*

8   To reiterate, consciousness itself is dynamic, attentive to both
     internal and external events in their full complexity, moment to
     moment.

9   Hufford summarizes an excellent example of this scientific/folk-
     loric approach when he reviews the work of Lehn and Schoreder
     who were able to explain merman sightings using ancient
     mariner's as well as scientific based data. The full reference is:
     Lehn, W.H., and Schroeder, I. (1981) The Norse Merman as an
     optical phenomenon. *Nature*, 289, 362-366.

10   In the references; Conesa 1995, 1997, 2000, and 2003

11   In the references; Conesa 2000

12   To this I would only add that different cultures' interpretation of
     The Old Hag experience, SP, because of language barriers and
     some unwillingness of the informants to share such a secret syn-
     drome, may be hard to come by, or, at first, the linguistic terms
     used to describe the universal events may be metaphors and words
     that need to be understood in the context of other descriptions
     Dr. Hufford refers to. See his point #5.

13   Percentages have varied depending on the population sampled,
     but I am confident that this number can be used generally as an
     estimate of its world-wide occurrence.

14   I use the terms 'hypnagogic' and 'hypnogogic' interchangeably.

15   I will side with Hufford on this claim but other researchers may
     disagree to the extent that SP correlates with emotional upheaval,
     extreme anxiety, and could be used as an indicator of significant
     deviations of normal routine that affect the dreamer detrimen-
     tally. Case in point, Firestone's demanding Newfoundlanders live
     in the fisheries with profound alterations of normal sleep cycles.
     Hufford was also correct in teasing out SP from narcolepsy proper,
     and other researchers have confirmed this.

16   Three-hour 'k' and 'aa' indices from the geomagnetic observatories in Ottawa and Victoria, Canada and in Fredericksburg, Virginia. These intensities were log 10 transformed as suggested by Delouis and Mayaud, 1975, and more recently by Dr. Coles.

Chapter One

17   I will be using, some may think abusing, the word 'uncanny' to stand for the SP/LD experience. I do this so that the non-SP experiencer does not take for granted the experiential import as 'spooky reality' of its phenomenology. Additionally the very term defined as something 'preternaturally strange' in Webster's New World Dictionary, helps to explain why the SP experience is treated as REAL.

18   Reasonable speculation is bound by the rules of what is 'likely' with present knowledge and, from our perspective, armed with the scientific method. Still I am dumbfounded at times by the double standards and application of 'reasonableness'. As a critical thinking exercise and example of the application of double standards while using reason I present my students with a fictional case where a raggedy, ignorant, filthy and half-crazed man, speaking with a thick and ancient accent, knocks on a believer's door, and claims to have heard the word of a god, and that this voice demands that the believer-respondent surrenders his/her only son for a sacrifice to the holy. Although most students say they would not heed this request nor think the man to be a representative of God, some of them nevertheless would accept a similar story and evidence as true and holy if it came sanctioned by authority. History and untested tradition makes just about anything respectable I suppose.

19   Aserinsky, E., and Kleitman, N. (1955) Two types of ocular motility occurring in sleep. *Journal of Applied Physiology*, 8 (1), 1-20. Aserinsky's observations of REM sleep began in 1951. See also Brown, C., 2003, *Smithsonian*, for a recent recounting of this early maverick in sleep research.

20   Two additional contributors to this foundational line of research were Nathaniel Kleitman, until his recent death, and William Dement, still an active sleep researcher at Stanford University.

21   *Microsomatognosia* is one of several somatognostic experiences (*Somatognosia*) that includes the feeling of flying and gliding—OBEs. Macrosomatognosia is the feeling of experiencing one's body or body parts as being unduly large.

22   Excluding conference presentations

23   Graduate and undergraduate students without a history of psychosis or narcolepsy

24   The area around the navel and the genitals has been related in many narrations of the experience as the locus of SP. In Chapter Five, meditation exercises for controlling SP make use of this observation.

25   This time span and present study might have broken the record as far as longitudinal studies of sleep/dreaming go, the previous one held and reported by Nathaniel Kleitman.

26   Richard Dawkins refers to the power and influence of culturally transmitted, useful, information as 'memes' in contrast to genetically transmitted information via genes.

Chapter Two

27   Our daughter is a very rational person and obviously has learned a lot from her papa about the physiology of sleep and dreaming but she still swears about the reality of these experiences.

28   Our daughter, might have inherited her condition also from my wife and her father and mother who experienced it frequently. In the case of my father-in-law he had the added environmental, occupational, aggravation of being a truck driver and losing REM sleep. He used to experience SP in conjunction with the altered schedules that come form long-haul driving.

29   Later on I will revisit Freud's concept of a *Hyper-Amnesic Dream* to illustrate that children, left on their own devices, manage the SP experience by interpreting it in a way that makes sense to them.

Of course, once an adult therapy has to unveil many layers and interpretations of an original SP experience.

30 Stewart, K (1969) Dream Theory in Malaya, In Charles T. Tart's (Editor) *Altered States of Consciousness*. Garden City, New York: Doubleday Anchor Book

31 In stories like the Holy Grail, Robin Hood, and Zen Koans, Wine, magical potions, forbidden fruits, and even sexual seduction may bring the traveler to a stupor that surely decides a demise and failure. Even Aladdin's three wishes are, when these expressed a wish to satisfy an immediate and banal desire, a test of wisdom, wisdom as delaying immediate gratification for a more encompassing and final truth.

32 Freud, S. (1900) *The Interpretation of Dreams* (Translated by A. A. Brill-1996). New York: Random House Value Publishing — Gracemercy Books—pp. 8-15

33 J. Piaget's lack of "object permanence," a milestone in human development when the baby appears to know that objects in her environment do not 'magically disappear' when they are removed from her sight.

34 See also Spanos et al., 1993: Close encounters: an examination of UFO experiences. *Journal of Abnormal Psychology*, 102, 624-632.

35 UFOs: Kidnapped by Aliens, produced by the Nova PBS series; A good media source and one of the last appearances by the late Carl Sagan in the role of the careful skeptic. I took his voice once or twice when writing about the probability of alien abduction.

Chapter Three

36 I used the word *comprehensive* deliberately because I believe that **SPS** also includes techniques that others have suggested (LaBerge) that may increase the probability of LD.

37 Susan Langer argues that dreams are examples of non-discursive expression.

38 With Mr. Robert Waggoner of The Lucid Dream Exchange; *www.dreaminglucid.com*. A comprehensive LD web site.

39 Theodore Roszak, in *The Voice of the Earth*; and Ralph Metzner, in *Green Psychology*

40 Langer, S. (1953) *Feeling and Form: A Theory of Art*. NY: Charles Scribner's Sons

41 Langer mentions several non-discursive principles that describe the processes of "mythic consciousness" (including Freud's *Over-determination* and *Ambivalence*) to be contrasted to the rules or principles that govern discursive logic such as "identity," "complementarity," and "excluded middle."

42 Langer, S. (1953) *Feeling and Form*, pp. 236-257.

43 This is Robert L. Van de Castle's approach also in "Our Dreaming Mind," 1994

44 Her position is generally accepted as a sign of mental stability for when insanity becomes the predominant force of the psyche then there is an erosion of *control* and ***purpose***. One can be slightly mad and very creative and society may look past the dysfunction. An example of this view might be the artist savants, though dysfunctional in many ways, can produce a restricted form of aesthetics.

45 This Haiku by the hermit Japanese Zen monk, Ryokan (1758-1831):

> ***The thief***
> ***Left it behind—***
> ***The moon and the window***

46 It is also true that time distortions occur during LD and story lines can seem to go on for a long time, in this sense the case for the phenomenological experience of LD and its psychological time makes it even more possible to creatively elaborate on dream content based on internally driven timelines.

47 Read about "Big" or Shamanic dreams in Chapter Four.

48 J.C.: The "roll up trick" was "taught" to me by an older and oriental lady while I was having a particularly distressing SP experience. She asked me to relax by breathing slowly and calmly, and then asked me to focus all my attention on my navel. As I did this I began to ***roll up as if I were a ball***. From there ***I entered a***

tunnel and ended up in a lucid dream. I call it the "roll up trick."
The same dream entity has offered and continues to offer further
advice with equal and practical results. Jorge, the scientist, has no
theory, hypothesis or explanation for the appearing entity other
than a weak and unconfirmed, "she must be an Anima construction of my unconscious". Yes, it sounds weak.

49   Ms. Gillis' hypothesis is elegant in every respect since in addition to being cognitively parsimonious still has a foothold on the
uncanny. I like it very much!

Chapter Four

50   Some sleep researchers have said this much, and I am forced
quarter after quarter to curtail their extreme reductionist rendition of dreaming in all my Psychology 100 courses.

51   The memory consolidation explanation for dreaming and the
above mentioned others do not address the complexity of dream
lucidity, self-awareness either. That is, memory consolidation is
a process that may not need self-awareness. For example, the
phenomenon of learning referred to as *kindling* operates at the
neuronal and unconscious level.

52   Neglectful, gracious or patronizing, either way, we go on having
lucid dreams

53   Being that nature and physiological processes operate under the
rule of "waste not", no neuronal process is truly random.

54   They are called "visions" or mystical experiences.

55   All of these practices, alone or in combination, have been used in
shamanism.

56   In the epilogue I propose a research question and hypothesis
consistent with the syncretic experiences of children being picked
up and carried by adults.

57   By logical extension, also, theories of consciousness that cannot
account for SP/LD are equally incomplete and perhaps even false.

58   Hobson tracks psychochemical waning and waxing functions
across three dimensions: 'A' Activation, 'I' Information flow, and

'M' the Mode of information processing. Presumably, any consciousness state can be mapped as a x,y,and z data points, *except for dream lucidity*.

59   SP still has a high value for functionality being the antithesis of mobility, hence my term "Bound Lucidity".

60   Negative as in a nightmare, positive as in a sex

61   Totally arbitrary on my part except that I was looking for an ascending number sequence that could be found in other naturally occurring events. However, a more appropriate measure—neuronal, physiological, and/or cognitive—needs to reflect actual, measurable movements along this space.

62   In Austin's *Zen and The Brain*, Table 9, pp. 300-303.

63   See in references, specifically the paper by Anderson, C. et al (1998) and the presentations by Takeshi Ieshima and Akifumi Tokosumi (1999).

64   To the subject

65   Shanon, B. (2003) Altered states and the study of consciousness—The case of Ayahuasca. *The Journal of Mind and Behavior*, Vol. 21, 2, pg. 145.

66   Unless of course the intake of hallucinogens is a daily or weekly practice and/or the shaman is so proficient in his/her conjuring that they can enter these states at will, at the drop of an Amazonian macaw plume.

Conclusion

67   Archetypal Psychology.

68   Even Freud warns about overanalyzing many dreams that convey obvious information. Their face value is enough.

69   Pages 347 through 428 in Brill's translation

70   Pages 364 through 376 in Brill's translation

71   In order not to think of this term diminutive translate "infantile" to original or to primal or to primitive or to animal.

72   As far as I know, no such place exists in our world geography, but if it did it would be located north of Imatra, in Finland. I made up

this location and ethnicity by combining the words *obligation* (as in paralysis) and *being* (as in becoming)= *Oblieng*. Sleep paralysis with lucid dreaming is thus the "obligated being" or one version of the shamanic experience.

Epilogue

73   Consistent with Freud's regression model, where strongly felt sensations and perceptions are relived during dreaming "discourse," a plausible hypothesis would be that the feeling of flying is associated with being carried by adults when we were children and moving, as though gliding, and perceiving this movement *syncretically*. That is, as an adult grasps our legs, thus bounded, we also have a high vantage point while this adult takes us down stairs or hillsides. The ambiguity of the sign we spoke about in earlier chapters is both about immobility and freedom. Interestingly, most accounts of "flying" during lucid dreaming are not of the fancy controlled F-16 type but more about gliding down at low altitudes with some restrictions placed on our mobility.

74   The idea and memory of a going through the birth canal has been proposed as well. I am equally interested in everyday and more prosaic circumstances that would impact dream content.

75   No a trivial matter for passing satellites.

Appendix I

Dream Event Classification and Description

Dream event classification expanded from Van Eeden (1913; 1918) and operational definitions for each dream type and category. The following definitions are also expanded from Conesa (1995) to include additional experiences or new dream events that occurred after the 1995 report, and later in the ten-year study as these demanded further clarifications or manifested themselves. These experiences are classified from states of no or little self-consciousness to a high degree of self-consciousness as illustrated in Figure 2.

No Dreams (ND): No memory of a dream exists in the morning after a night of sleep nor a later recollection of a dream makes an appearance. After one such dreamless night, I would respond to a inquiry such as "Did you dream last night?" with an adamant "I had no dreams last night." Nor a memory of a past dream will be remembered at a later occasion (see definition for a "reminiscence" below).

Flimsies (FS): Flimsies are akin to a "tip-of-the-tongue" phenomena; one is sure something was dreamt but one cannot retrieve the information. There might have been a negative emotional tone associated with a dream not remembered, hence this is one of the reasons that it permeates through consciousness, that continues as uneasiness and unsettledness.

A reminiscence (R): Experientially, they start out like no-dreams except that during the day, and while awake, a certain image, event, object, situation, triggers a vague or clear recollection of some image, event, object, situation that occurred in a dream usually the night before. Thus a *reminiscence* is more like regular dream except that it is not remembered unless a contextual cue occurs after awakening.

Regular Dreams (RD): Unlike dreams with a major and definable visual component, these tend to be less developed and more vague than vivid or lucid dreams. Most of the time, and upon awakening, there is only the certainty that one had a dream accompanied by a brief emotion, perceptual image and the last words of a sentence. I logged my regular dreams, as imperfect, fuzzy, black and white images that include one or mode scenes. Generally, there is little story elaboration or decipherable context associated with these fleeting recollections.

Vivid Dreams (VD): These dreams are rich in sensorial detail, often as lucid dreams are. They are characterized as having elaborate and well-defined stories, in recognizable behavioral, psychological, or social contexts, and explicitly adhere to understandable, even predictable, plots. Emotions can be felt as deeply as in complex awake situations. A lot of nightmares and dreams with a sexual component fall into this category, more precisely, the negative content, N (-), and the sexual content, SX, dream events. However, and in contrast with negative or sexual themes in lucid dreams, there is not a self-aware "I" controlling the events occurring in the dream, only an observer who reacts to dream situations in unpredictable ways (Hartmann, 1984). As explained in Chapter X, this category includes dreams with sexual content and nightmares.

Extra Vivid Dreams (XV): Vivid dreams that crossed an experiential threshold of degree of *cognitive embeddedness*, as described in Chapter X, and were not lucid dreams—there was no intense sense of self-awareness or degree of control— became dream events of this type. The justification, one that was necessary after the fifth year of data collection, for this additional class of dream events came about when vivid dreams were "about something" or repeated themselves, a recurring vivid dream, or, more importantly, where highly detailed information was obtained in a vivid dream. Another way to describe their experiential import is to say that they "impose" themselves onto the dreamer, or that a sense of emergency in conveying a particular kind of information is evident tied to a particular piece of information. The informational "imposition" was more cognitive-perceptual than sensorial. That is, the information received had a cognitive structure that demanded higher order cognitive processes—in contrast to sensorial processes—that included focused and selective attention, memorization and recollection, evaluation of emotional tone and appropriately responding to this tone. Extra vivid dreams, because of their cognitive and impositional nature, were as impacting, and in many cases even more so, than SPs or LDs. These were rare events, 33 in all as compared to the reported 839 vivid dreams.

Lucid Dreams (LD): Lucid dreams are dreams with a high degree of self-awareness, within which one feels that one is fully conscious. One has the certainty that one is dreaming while in the midst of a dream. Usually, in such a dream, there is conscious and verbal formulation of statements such as, "How about that, I am dreaming!" Volition—deciding how the dream progresses, or moving from dream to dream— and control—if flying, aptly maneuvering the dreaming-body, or controlling functions such as speed— are also common features of these dreams (LaBerge, 1980; Gackenback, 1991). There is a tendency to control the dream in ways that defy physical laws. For example, floating, gliding or flying-lucid dreams are very common. Common also are dreams where one's stride is antigravitational, leaping effortlessly about. Because the lucid dreamer possesses volition and control in a lucid dream one is also empowered to control further dream elements and situations and also to pursue lucid dreaming again as a methodology of dreaming. Lucid dreams are usually vivid, almost always in color (for me) and rich in detail. Music is sometimes heard and played with a great degree of richness and surrealism, beyond what real music would sound like (ethereal). In lucid dreams that incorporate me playing an instrument, it usually happens that the composition is original and that the music persists even after awaking. While in a lucid dream is not uncommon to be standing in front of (or interacting with) an aesthetically beautiful object, including paintings, flowers, birds, jewels, expanses of grass, stairs, blocks of granite or marble, trees, gold, rocks, water, and even the soft skin or fur of another entity. Additionally, lucid dreams involve the manipulation of energy (bands, balls, serpentines) by massaging it, throwing it, and making it do some other specific maneuver.

Sleep Paralysis (SP): These usually predormital events occur when dreamers find themselves fully conscious struggling out of an atonic state and incapable of producing speech. Dreamers report hearing strange sounds like buzzing; booms with pain in their neck, head or abdomen; crackling; ringing; or electrical-like feelings running through their bodies hours, minutes before or during the SP episode. Hypnogogic hallucinations are sometimes reported as part of the SP episode which include a feeling of oppression on the chest and a difficulty with breathing. Hufford (1982) distinguishes, and phenomenological reports confirm it, between these states, because they can occur independently of each other. Through the years the author and other individuals develop methods for waking up from the paralysis state or to move into lucid dreaming (see SPS). In order to awaken from SP the experiencer works out a signal with his/her sleeping partner that helps him or her wake up and out of the paralysis. These signals included slight finger movements or moans to be interpreted as "wake me up."

Hypnogogic Hallucinations (HH): Is REM dreaming and dreaming material experienced with lucidity and self-awareness at *sleep onset*. They can occur alone or in conjunction with SP symptoms. Sometimes reported as part of the SP experience.

Hypnopompic Hallucinations (HP): Is REM dreaming and dreaming material experienced with lucidity and self-awareness while *waking from a dream*. They can occur alone and less frequently reported in conjunction with SP symptoms.

Hallucination (H): Under unusual conditions, and as part of the rituals of preparing to go to bed, subjects have reported what they referred to as visions, when they knew that they were not asleep. Please refer to a full description of this event in Chapter Two.

Other Dream Events and Dream Event Qualifiers

The Nightmare

Unfortunately for the dream researcher, the term Nightmare is both a dream type and a negative emotional qualifier for other dream events to the extent that most people use the term to refer to a very bad and intense dream (the same duality and ambiguity occurs Spanish term, Pesadilla). In this sense, the term nightmare is very imprecise for a scientific study unless it can be operationalized and given an universal sign meaning. Folklore studies of SP usually begin with an attention to any anthropological reference to "bad dreams" because it may be the case that field investigators generically translate these as a nightmare. In my ten-year report I refer to nightmares as Negative Content dreams, N(-), and are different from HH or HP experiences such as the incubus. Elsewhere in the literature as Hufford observes, Nightmares are of two types. One is associated with the SP experience and includes usually a hypnagogic hallucination. This experience is identical to the older definition and experience of nightmare, or incubus. In such cases there might an actual attack by a singular entity, a variety of beings, actual touching be unseen hands, or even the feeling of a sinister entity or presence (FOP) lurking about in the bedroom.

Flying

The feeling of flying can occur in a vivid, extra vivid, or in a lucid dream. It sometimes occurs when an SP experiencer gains control of his/her paralysis condition and "wills" "flying" from the belly area. In such cases, the SP experiencer may first experience being compressed, or squeezed through a tunnel space, cavities, ribbons, or before they can "fly". Variations of actual dream flying include experiences of gliding, floating, raising gently, walking or running effortless in big leaps.

Out-of-body Experiences

An out-of-body experience, OBE, is the cognitive realization that there is a sort of dream-body that exists independently from the sleeping, physical body. This is confirmed when the experiencer "sees" his/her physical body lying in his/her bed while he/she floats about in their bedrooms. Additional confirmation comes when the dreamer is able to bump into objects; look at very fine details of objects and textures thought to be present in the bedroom. This realization occurs with intense self-awareness. As reported in the text, OBEs can and do occur, sometimes in conjunction with the very first SP experience and in subsequent events. During the ten years of official recording SP episodes there were four OBEs that occurred in the same night as when an SP occurred, preceded an SP, or followed it. Equally, an OBE experience can turned in flying, gliding, standing, dragging oneself on the ground with great effort, floating, or raising gently. Interestingly, and in contrast to "flying" experiences, OBEs are rarely about walking.

Tunnels, Spins, and Drains

As mentioned before, while in the grip of SP, sometimes it is possible to spontaneously or by choice, "wriggle out" of the paralysis by means of pushing, traveling, or crawling through, in a tight space reported as a tunnel, a corridor, tight clothing—sleeping bags included-, or the implosion of one's own body. The SPS methodology includes recognizing that while in SP one can divert one's attention to an area of one's body, typically, the navel region, in order to purposely experience the spinning and going through the tunnel. This sensation is not unlike a feeling of being sucked and at the same time shrunk or made flexible in order to fit through the tunnel. There is a similarity between these experiences and the shamanic journey anthropologist Michael Harner reports. For example he says, "Entrances into the Lowerworld commonly lead down into a tunnel or tube that conveys the shaman to an exit, which opens out upon bright and marvelous landscapes." He specifically cites the experiences of an Iglulik shaman as, "He almost glides as if as falling through a tube so fitted to his body that he can check his progress by pressing against the sides," or the account of a Tavgi Samoyed shaman, "As I looked around, I noticed a hole in the earth. The hole became larger and larger. We descended through it and arrived at a river with two streams flowing in opposite directions."

APPENDIX II

SP Symptoms

Somatosensory, vestibular, and other phenomena associated with sleep paralysis (SP) and lucid dreaming (LD). Like in Appendix I, the following descriptions and classifications have been expanded from the 1995 study to include the entire ten years and the accounts of other subjects.

Perceived as Exo-somatic but Affecting the Body

Waves, vibrations, electrical-like currents, and earthquake-like tremors (SP)—Hours or minutes preceding the SP episode.

Acoustic-like

Non-entity, non-human: Crackling, snapping, buzzing, ringing, booms (booming)—Hours or minutes preceding the SP episode.

Human-like, entity-like: Voices saying (whispering, shouting, saying) specific words, phrases understood by the dreamer—commanding, beckoning, supplicating, screaming, or threatening the dreamer; animal-like moans, groans, growls.

Musical: Music is sometimes heard or produced with great richness and surreal, sound quality. Myself and other subjects have reported listening to and/or composing songs or instrumental pieces that can be remembered and hummed to upon awakening (see also Van Eeden, 1913; 1918). These experiences can occur during LDs but not exclusively. Additionally, myself and other subjects report playing unusual instruments, never seen before, stringed or winds, or playing an instrument for which they have no training.

Visual-like

General: The perception that occurs while in an OBE episode, that the lighting quality is eternally dusk, or purple, or blue-gray. Also, this category includes the perception and interaction with luminous blobs (blue, red, orange, pink or amber light); seeing auras; the almost microscopic perception of objects and details of wall, ceiling, or bed lining (crevices, surface textures, and x-ray see through vision)—SP. During the LD experience, this translates into the perception of vibrant and/or surreal colors. Seeing otherworldly beings in the bedroom, particularly, hands reaching for the dreamer.

Sleep Paralysis

Complete or partial body atonia. Also, in LDs is these are connected to SPs, the feeling of immobility or heaviness that prevent the dreamer from moving about.

Somatosensoty

This category includes rotation of the body (pivot: the belly area), twisting of the body, rolling into oneself, and spinning. Also, pressure on different parts of the body, but most commonly on the chest and belly area, flying, gliding, floating, hovering, and being squeezed through diverse versions of a narrow tubular aperture such as tunnels. Pain in various parts of the body but usually reported on different locations of the trunk and belly.

Microsomatognosia: The feeling of shrinking in size until a

JORGE CONESA SEVILLA, PH.D.

perceived body crumbles into a ball or small form, or the perception of other normal size objects and entities (including other humans) as being small in size (from one to three feet).

Macrosomatognosia: The feeling of growing in size, less common than Microsomatognosia, or the perception, more frequent, of other objects and entities as being twice to three times their normal size.

Dissociation: Out-of-body experiences, or the feeling that a dreaming-body is independent from a physical body.

Hypnogogic Hallucinations

Perceiving out of the ordinary and intense realities during sleep onset (predormital). Specific to the SP phenomena these hallucinations includes numerous, trans-cultural, and historical reports that fall under repeatable patterns illustrated in the older meaning of "nightmare" as an "Old Hag," a malignant female presence; an "Incubus," or a male entity—spirit or demon— visiting a female dreamer for the purposes of having sexual intercourse; and/or the "Succubus" the female counterpart of the Incubus seeking sexual contact with a male dreamer for the same purpose. The Incubus and Succubus experiences also include a feeling of pressure, a physical burden, generalized oppression, and immobility. Sometimes also, the feeling of being touched, pulled, caressed, or being in physical contacted with a hallucinated entity. The commonalities of these experiences across cultures and their specific descriptions allows for a scientific study of the SP experience unlike the multifaceted phenomenology associated with other dream events and phenomenology.

Hypnopompic Hallucinations: Perceiving out of the ordinary and intense realities while waking up (postdormital). Same experiences as in hypnagogic hallucinations but lacking in frequency the experience of a succubus or incubus.

Other

"Bolt of Lightning" exploding at the base of the neck and spreading thought the head and body in waves and accompanied by auditory hallucinations listed above. This bolt of lightning can be described as "snake-like" as the sensation weaves through the different body parts. Its final "expulsion" form the body is usually accompanied by vivid dream imagery and lucid dreams.

APPENDIX III

Case Studies: SP/LD Full-length Narratives

The following are verbatim excerpts from several case studies except for grammatical errors corrected by author ("torsil"=torso; "violent"=violently; also, parentheses clarifications are mine) and were taken from narrative studies. These excerpts are thus from the fifty narratives reported in Conesa (2000) and from a larger data set. Overall, females report SP episodes in greater detail and are more open to share but male and females incidences are equal. When pertinent, I have added additional comments between the brackets.

Case "JB," male, 24
"a feeling of being stuck to my bed and I can't move . . . the floating . . . I felt my feet begin to rise, and then my head, but my torso remained on the bed and then my whole body began to tremble with fear and then I was released and I woke up drenched in sweat . . . I felt myself being dragged around the room very, very fast and violently, but the room was empty . . . I sense an evil spirit doing the dragging . . . I heard a male voice and it was coming from the ceiling and it said, 'It's time to play games now.' I strained to get up and finally I did. I got something to drink and went back to sleep but I was very scared. The other voice during another episode was a female voice and it said, 'What are you going to do (JC)."

Case "CM," male, 27

"a warping of my current surroundings" [sleeping position: laying on stomach, head slightly elevated by a pillow and facing either left or right]

Case "RT," male, 19

"building of electricity in my head . . . When I had SP the next day, I relaxed and went through the extremely uncomfortable transition (electricity), but once I was asleep, man was it worth it. I can't even begin to describe the lucidity and my ability to create whatever I wanted, have it just as clear as reality, and remember every single detail—I FLEW myself around campus—"

Case "CM2,"

" . . . it never happens when I wake up its when I go to sleep, one second I'm lying thinking, and the next thing I can't move, I seem to be breathing heavily, sometimes I seem to be floating or flying, and I get a weird sensation of buzzing though me . . . sometimes I am half dreaming as well and someone is pinning me down or something, or there is somebody in the room with me . . . " [sleeping position: laying on stomach, facing left]

Case "KG," female, forties

"For years, I have experienced the phenomenon of sleep paralysis, but not knowing what it was, I called it 'my ghost'. I would awaken and be fully aware but unable to move because of an oppressive spirit—which felt completely evil—sitting on my back and pressing down on me. I was certain it was trying to posses me, and all I could do was to lie still and wait for it to go away...Sometimes, and out-of-body experience accompanied these dreams. Other times, I felt I was being sucked up into some sort of a cloud" [NIGHT MARCHERS—Tunnels-circle of clouds]

Case "E," female, 61

" (I) remember the first dream paralysis I had, was 13 and moved to a new house. I have it all now not as bad . . . pressure on body, cannot move, open eyes, see room but cannot move . . . screaming and wondering if my husband can hear me of if nothing is coming out, trying to move, that when I wake up am exhausted . . . loud humming noise in my head, and I think am going to have a heart attack its so loud . . . also felt someone putting a pillow on my face and helpless. I think the worse is feeling someone next to me pressing against."

Case "NM," male, 23

"I get a buzzing feeling in my head . . . a few minutes later I can't move with terrible pains going though my body, sometimes with hallucinations PP. This happens just as I'm about to fall asleep"

Case "DS," male, 39

[Explanation of present life situation/circumstances generating high anxiety and turmoil, thinking that they may be contributing to his SP episodes]

"I kept thinking/dreaming that there was someone in my apartment and was going to be hurt or killed at any instant. I dreamt at least four times of rising from the bed and going and checking the front door, with the dread and feeling that I was confronting an evil by doing so." [social anxiety connected to recent events]

Case "JG," female

"I experience the suffocation feeling, as well as the 'hissing' for lack of a better explanation, on top of my head, which is painful as well. I can usually shake myself out in minutes, but if I try to go to sleep without getting up and moving around for awhile, it will occur almost immediately after the first . . . (these episodes) do happen more frequently when I lie on my back." [an example of a coping technique]

Case "S," female

I have been experiencing SP for a long time, My family has too. I found it weird that some did, and others did not. I have attacks when I am on my back or any position . . . My senses grow very acute when I am having an attack. My attacks are painful, there is a feeling of drilling, sawing, buzzing, etc felt all over my body. It's painful. My attacks last about a minute or two and when I wake up I am so exhausted and my heart is racing like a locomotive . . . I really do not dream when I have an attack, its like the confusion going on darkness, static screens like on a TV. or something. I had one the other morning, . . . I wiggle my fingers and my face and I fell out of it." [familial and coping technique]

Case "G," female, 26 [a rich and canonical example: it includes a familial history, vortex, with coping strategies]

"I have had SP for about five years and my dad also has it when he was younger. I began having SP in college. The first time it happened, I dreamed that I was flying toward a large vortex. As I got close to it, however, I got scared and didn't want to go inside. When I tried to turn back, the scene changed. I was now flying/falling—but it was really happening, I really felt like I was falling. I could hear a loud buzzing in my ears and it became violently windy. (they happen—SP) shortly after I fall asleep, after I've been up late . . . then I usually have the sensation that I am beginning to float out of my body, except for some reason I never have a full 'out of body experience' . . . feel my body vibrating . . . do feel the feeling of presence sometimes but usually is just perceive as some invisible thing touching me, or trying to pull me out of my body, and it is not really malevolent—just there . . . one time, and this is actually kind of funny, I 'woke up' and these little people about two feet high dragged me out of bed and onto the floor. I really thought that I was on the floor, but after I got out of the paralysis and really woke up, I was in my bed....if I go back to sleep right away, it will happen two, three or four times. it always happens when I am lying on my back...(a different SP episode) when I looked up there was this huge beast with its front legs on the end of my bed. It was black and four feet tall. Probably four feet long too. It was muscular—very big. But what I remember the most is its teeth. It had these huge teeth and growled at me. I couldn't move. It came up onto my bed at me and growled and breathed on me. I remember its breath was very heavy. I made the sign of the cross in my mind. Although I am not religious, I was raised Catholic and it was about the only thing I could think to do at that point. It snarled at me one last time and those teeth came at me—about a foot from my face. I could feel its breath. Then it disappeared. I struggled out of the paralysis fairly quickly and woke up."

Case "MR", male, 16

"Recently, for the first time, I experienced what I think you described as dream paralysis. I awoke from sleeping (well I thought I did) with my face right in front of this plastic spinning coil I have suspended from my fan over my bed in my room. I thought I had awoken and decided to throw myself on my back, onto my bed. I did this, and slowly floated down onto my bed, that scared the hell out of me. Once I landed in my body my nuts (yes my crotch) started to sink intensely into the bed. I had the strangest sensation in my groin, of it just being pulled into the bed, and then I woke up".

Case "AJ", [Relating experiences about sister and mother: familial]

"My sister experienced one (SP) last night and another one a few months before that. My mother has been plagued by them for years."

Case "W", female [spouse disbelief, feels alone, cannot communicate her SP]

"After last night having such a disturbing episode and trying to explain it to my spouse I found myself searching on the net for some answers...First of all, I have been suffering this for years. Sometimes I have as many as three or four attacks in one night or it will leave for a couple of months...(SPs occur) when I doze off to sleep, but it can happen when I am in the middle of sleep...(the first thing that happens) is I feel as if my brain is asleep like you would a limb like an arm or leg it is very uncomfortable and all you know is that you have to wake up... I (am also) aware of sounds and light and people, sometimes I can actually see things. I have learned to wake myself up while swinging my arms, which feel like anchors are tied to them, and flipping my head around to wake up. Sometimes I am able to let out a moan. I'm trying to say "help me" but I can't move my lips."

Case "SC", female, 29 [spouse disbelief, cannot communicate her SP, and is a nurse: occupational factor of SP]

"I am a RN...Its weird, I have not told anyone but my spouse about these sensations (until yesterday) because I thought I either was psycho, had some pretty wild dreams, or had spirits following me...My most recent occurrence happened over the past weekend (May 9th to be exact)...that night I was asleep on my left side when I felt a sudden severe pain, like something was crushing my head. I tried to move but my body was paralyzed. I tried to yell to wake up my husband, but all I could do was moan, because I couldn't even move my mouth. It (SP) let up and I had a minute or two of relaxation before it started again. The same things occurred, I couldn't move my lips or my body. I remember seeing that I was laying on my left side, seeing my husband lying next to me, knowing well where I was, so I didn't think I was dreaming. After that, I woke up my husband, who said it was probably just a dream, but I was too terrified to go back to sleep. I wouldn't even get up to go to the bathroom, until daylight. I mentioned it to a physician I work with yesterday, and he said it sounds like sleep paralysis."

Case "KO", female, 34 [feels she is alone with her SP situation, a highly intelligent individual, sexual assault of entity]

"I have suffered from sleep paralysis for about 10 years. I never knew until this week that THIS WAS AN ACTUAL TERM for what I experience several times a year, and have never told anyone about! I am amazed. I thought it was something very weird, but although I am educated and intelligent, I did not realize it was a diagnosed occurrence. My experiences with SP always includes 2 "entities", a malevolent male (who, to be blunt, usually, sexually penetrates me and brings me to orgasm) and a female who lurks behind."

Case "LL", female

"I have been having lucid dreams as long as I can remember. I have them almost every night. But about a year ago I began having sleep paralysis, approximately once every three or four weeks on average…My most recent sleep paralysis episode was about two weeks ago, although I don't keep a journal so I don't remember the exact date. I do remember it occurred just before 4:40 AM Pacific time in . . . , California . . . I had the feeling there were vampires after me and they were trying to sneak into my room through cracks where the ceiling meets the walls. Second, I felt like someone was tightening a belt around my stomach, supposedly for the purpose of keeping the vampires away, although I kept saying that doing so made no sense whatsoever. Because I was afraid, I tried to astral project out of my body, but what ended up happening was that I floated, paralyzed, from the bed up to the ceiling, and felt very distinctly the sharpness of the stucco against my exposed skin (I was fully clothed in pajamas as I slept, but in the dream I was naked). I could see the stucco too, in great detail. This episode was the scariest I've ever had and it took a long time for me to fully wake up and come out of the state. When I did, I walked around my apartment".

Case "BB"

"One night, as I was sleeping in my sister's bedroom, I experience paralysis and what I think was probably a lucid dream. Before I fell asleep that night, I had been thinking about aliens because I was sleeping next to a giant Pink Floyd poster with a very scary face on it. I fell asleep freaked out. Then, suddenly I was "looking around the room" and was "looking at the poster on the wall" and I was telling myself to wake up. Then, during this, I realized that I couldn't move and I thought I was being abducted or something. I was lying on my stomach, and I couldn't turn over and I remember my arm being next to me and I just couldn't move it. In a panic, I tried to scream "help me," and I was trying so hard to speak-I can't remember putting forth that much effort ever before, I started to shake and a little noise came out and then, all of a sudden, rather abruptly, I could move again. So then I jumped up and ran out of the room. But it was so scary. It hasn't happened to me since."

APPENDIX IV

Shamanic Dreaming Cube Reality Index

(By Jorge Conesa ©)

Name _____ Sex ___ Age _____ Ethnicity _____
Classify Dream event using Appendix I _____

For instructions on how to score this questionnaire please go to the end of this appendix.

[Note to the reader: subjects do not see the headings for these dimensions, and the questions within each dimension can be randomized for factor analytic purposes. Neither do subjects see the number weights affixed to each item, e.g., "Flying 3". In keeping with the nomenclature of the Dreaming Cube, some of the emotional items in Section C have positive or negative valences.]

A. Functional Control

Please check a box indicating if the particular action, behavior, or situation took place in your dream. You can select as many boxes as necessary in order to describe all the events that transpired in your dream.

- ☐ Flying 3
- ☐ Controlled flying 5
- ☐ Walking 5

- ☐ Standing 1
- ☐ Standing but moving other body parts 2
- ☐ Standing but tense 2
- ☐ Paralyzed in a dream 2
- ☐ Lethargic in a dream 2
- ☐ Paralyzed in my bed, but not in a dream 5
- ☐ Lethargic, but not in a dream but while trying to wake up from a dream 1
- ☐ My "legs felt as if they were lead" in a dream 3
- ☐ Fighting 3
- ☐ Dancing 4
- ☐ Gliding 3
- ☐ Controlled gliding 5
- ☐ Hovering 3
- ☐ Controlled hovering 5
- ☐ Sitting in meditation 4
- ☐ Sitting in meditation and experiencing a peaceful or Satori moment 5
- ☐ Manipulating an object with your hands, feet, legs, arms, or any other body part 5
- ☐ Eating 4
- ☐ Having intercourse willingly 5
- ☐ Being forced to have intercourse 4
- ☐ Talking 3
- ☐ Singing 5
- ☐ Reading 4
- ☐ Writing 5

Please include any other activity not mentioned in this list or qualify (expand) any of the questions to include additional information:

_____

_____

_____

B. Perceptual Acuity

Please check a box indicating the particular perception, sensation, or percept witnessed or manipulated in your dream. You can select as many boxes as necessary in order to describe all the events that transpired in your dream.

- ☐ Black and white scenes 2
- ☐ I dreamt in color 4
- ☐ I dreamt both in color and in black and white 4
- ☐ Images seemed blurry in my dream 1
- ☐ I was able to feel a particular texture (soft, rough, prickly, slimy, etc.) 4
- ☐ I saw a distinct face (or faces) that I could recognize on the street 4
- ☐ I saw a distinct face (or faces) that I could not recognize on the street 3
- ☐ I saw colors and these were very intense and sharp 5
- ☐ I saw brilliant objects 6
- ☐ I was able to read text 5
- ☐ I heard music or other sounds distinctly 4
- ☐ I felt pain 5
- ☐ I gave or received a kiss and felt it 5
- ☐ I felt pleasurable sensations 4
- ☐ I felt sexual pleasure and felt my genitalia participate in the sexual act 4
- ☐ I felt sexual pain when my genitalia participated in a forced sexual act 4
- ☐ I was able to smell an object in my dream 7
- ☐ I was able to taste an object in my dream 7
- ☐ Someone was touching me in my dream 4
- ☐ I saw a distinct pattern, new or familiar to me 5
- ☐ I experienced depth (three dimensionality) 7
- ☐ I could move about in three dimensions 6

☐ This dream was as real as everyday reality 7
☐ This dream was more real than everyday reality 7

Please include any other activity not mentioned in this list or qualify (expand) any of the questions to include additional information:

_____

_____

_____

C. Intensity of Emotion

Please check a box indicating the degree and the type of emotion felt. You can select as many boxes as necessary in order to describe all the events that transpired in your dream.

☐ This was a bad dream -1
☐ This was a very bad dream -2
☐ This was a nightmare -3
☐ This was a neutral dream 0
☐ This was a good dream +1
☐ This was a very good dream +2
☐ This was a blissful experience and dream +3
☐ I cried in my dream + or - 2
☐ I laughed in my dream +2
☐ I hated someone in my dream -3
☐ I felt rage in my dream -4
☐ I felt anger in my dream -4
☐ I felt pleasure in my dream +4
☐ I felt protected and secure in my dream +2
☐ I felt that someone was after me in my dream + or - 3
☐ I was being chased by someone or something and I was afraid -4

- ☐ Something or someone was sitting on my chest and I was afraid -6
- ☐ Something or someone was in my room and I was afraid -5
- ☐ Something or someone was sitting on my chest but I was not afraid 6
- ☐ Something or someone was in my room but I was not afraid 5
- ☐ I felt guilty in my dream -2
- ☐ I killed someone in self-defense but I still felt badly -3
- ☐ I felt little emotion in my dream 1
- ☐ I felt no emotion in my dream 0

Please include any other activity not mentioned in this list or qualify (expand) any of the questions to include additional information:

_____

_____

_____

D. Cognitive Embeddedness: Quality and Degree of Information Obtained

Please check a box indicating the degree to which you interacted with dream objects, persons, or environment. Obviously, because this is an evaluation of the quality of dream content, even if the question does not say "in my dream" assume it. You can select as many boxes as necessary in order to describe all the transactions that transpired in your dream.

- ☐ I carried on a conversation and remembered everything that was said 5
- ☐ I remember the specific words that were said 6
- ☐ I did math in my dream 6
- ☐ I interacted with a person to the same degree of interaction as awake 6

- ☐ A dream entity provided practical instructions that were useful in my dream 7
- ☐ A dream entity provided practical instructions that were useful while awake 7
- ☐ None of the instructions that a dream entity provided were practical or useful 5
- ☐ I held an object in my hand and was able to study it at length 4
- ☐ I interacted with a person or animal I knew had died 4
- ☐ I interacted with a person or animal who I knew to be alive 4
- ☐ I interacted with an animal and the animal shared information with me 5
- ☐ I interacted with a vague and ghostly entity who shared information with me 5
- ☐ I wrestled with a ghost for what seemed to be minutes in my bedroom 7
- ☐ I wrestled with a hairy beast for what seemed to be minutes in my bedroom 7
- ☐ I faced a billboard or announcement and was able to read it 5
- ☐ I had to pull off leech-type creatures attached to my body and skin 6
- ☐ I found myself on what seemed to be another planet 5
- ☐ I could change my dreams at will 8
- ☐ I could travel between different dreams at will 9
- ☐ I played a musical instrument and remember the melody or the lyrics 6
- ☐ I was teaching others to manipulate objects in my dream 5
- ☐ I was teaching others how to fly in my dream 6
- ☐ I was guided by blobs of light to pursue other dreams 8
- ☐ I was taken by blobs of light to pursue other dreams 7
- ☐ I was asked by blobs of light to follow them to pursue other dreams 9

Please include any other activity not mentioned in this list or qualify (expand) any of the questions to include additional information:

_____

_____

_____

Scoring

As explained before in Chapter Four, the "vividness" of a dream is a function of the higher numerical ranking obtained from the items in each dimension. Obviously, lucid dreaming with control is the highest ranking and most vivid dream experience. Therefore, any item that triangulates toward lucid dreaming is valued higher. For that reason more items in Section D, in general, have been given this highest ranking. Additionally, and for the same reason, Section A is also valued higher. That means that obtaining a higher score in sections B and C with lower scores in A and D diagnoses a vivid dream but not as vivid as a lucid dream. An example of this would be experiencing night terrors or waking from a nightmarish dream with little recollection of dream content. One can argue further that most negative dreams are so labeled precisely because the dreamer is defenseless in a given situation, under threat, and with little capacity to change dream events: a victim rather than a willful dreamer. So controlling any aspect of dreaming is ranked higher across all of the sections.

Moreover, given my own experience and the independent comments and experiences of other lucid dreamers, one can claim that there is a developmental progression from sections A-C leading into Section D. In this sense, Section D is a shamanic outcome of sorts provided sufficient dreaming control is achieved, extreme emotional sets are under the control of the dreamer, and paralysis is surmounted and later used as a spring board for greater "dream embeddedness."

Seasoned SP and/or LD experiencers allude to or explicitly comment on this progression.

The numerical rankings for each item were averaged from hundreds of volunteered dream reports and from my own experiences. Subjects did not know that I was coding and ranking their narratives so I suspect that they were naive with respect to their input and final use. For example, an outcome of this data gathering is that "Walking" in Section A is ranked higher than "Flying." But as many lucid dreamers know, walking is a more rare dream event, especially walking with control and ease of mobility, than flying because it implies the coordination of more body parts than simply darting through dream space.

Having obtained a score from a subject (for example: A= 55; B= 32; C= +40; C= 100) one can begin to assess the experiential quality of any dream event in a manner that leads to quantification. By the way, depending on the overwhelming effect and emotion of a dream, it can usually be designated as a neutral, positive or negative dream. However, some dreams may include all three emotional states in which case the "C" score has three parts and values.

Finally, one can then plot these data inside a dreaming cube and visually compare this dream event to another from the same person or to the dream events and experiences of other dreamers.

A final caveat, this questionnaire is admittedly a fairly new tool and I have not normalized its use. Although it contains enough face validity because it emerged from many narratives and contributions, it needs to be tested with larger samples to be sure. The items in any of the sections can be changed, or additional sections can be added to focus on other aspects of dream content.

BIBLIOGRAPHY AND REFERENCES

Allport, G.W. (1955) Becoming: basic considerations for a psychology of personality. New Haven and London: Yale University Press.(pp.87.)

Aserinsky, E., and Kleitman, N. (1955) Two types of ocular motility occurring in sleep. *Journal of Applied Physiology*, 8, 1, 1-20.

Asmara-Winang, B. Tindihan in Indonesia. Personal Communication.

Austin, J.H. (1999) Zen and the brain: toward an understanding of meditation and consciousness. Cambridge, MA: MIT Press.

Baars, B.J. (1988) A cognitive theory of consciousness. NY: Cambridge University Press.

Baars, B., Newman, J., & Taylor, J. (1998) Neuronal mechanisms of consciousness: A Relational Global Workspace framework. In S. Hameroff, A. Kaszniak, and J. Laukes, (Eds.), Toward a Science of Consciousness II: The second Tucson discussions and debates. Cambridge, MA: MIT Press.

Belisheva, N.K., Popov, A.N., Petukhova, N.V., Pavlova, L.P., Osipov, K.S., Tkachenko, S.E., Baranova, T.I. (1995) Qualitative and quantitative evaluation of the effects of geomagnetic field variations on the functional state of the human brain. *Biophysics*, 40, 1007-1014.

Bell, C.C., Shakoor, B., Thomson, B. (et al.) (1984) Prevalence of isolated sleep paralysis in black students. *J. Natl. Med. Ass.*, 76, 501-508.

Bell, C.C., Dixie-Bell, D.D., B., Thomson, B. (1986) Further studies on the prevalence of isolated sleep paralysis in black students. *J. Natl. Med. Ass.*, 78, 649-659.

Bell, C.C., Hildreth, C.J., Jenkins, E.J., Carter, C. (1988) The relationship of isolated sleep paralysis and panic disorder to hypertension. *J. Natl. Med. Ass.*, 80, 289-294.

Binns, E. (1842) The anatomy of sleep: or the art of procuring sound and refreshing slumber at will. London: John Churchill.

Blackmore, S. (1982) *Beyond the Body*. London: Heinemann.

Blackmore, S. (1984) A psychological theory of the out-of-body experience. *Journal of Parapsychology*, 48, 201-218.

Blackmore, S. (1991) Lucid Dreaming: Awake in you sleep? *Skeptical Inquirer*, 15, 362-370.

Blackmore, S. (1998) Abduction by aliens or sleep paralysis? *Skeptical Inquirer*, 22, 3.

Brugger, P. (1994) Are "presences" preferentially felt along the left side of one's body? *Perceptual and Motor Skills*, 79, 1200-1202.

Brugger, P. (1996) Unilaterally felt "presences": the neuropsychiatry of one's invisible Doppleganger *Neuropsychiatry, Neuropsychology, and Behavioral Neurology*, 2, 114-122.

Buchler, J. (1955) The philosophy of Peirce: Selected writings. New York: Routledge and Kegan Paul Ltd.

Brown, C. (2003) The stubborn scientist who unraveled a mystery of the night. *Smithsonian*, October 2003, 92-100.

Calvo, C. (1995) The three halves of Ino Moxo: Teachings of the wizard of the upper Amazon. (Translation by Kenneth A. Symington). Vermont: Inner traditions International.

Campbell, J. (1988) The Power of myth. In Betty Sue Flowers (ed.) John Campbell The Power of Myth with Bill Moyers. New York: Doubleday.

Carroll, R. Night Marchers in Hawaii. Personal Communication.

Cohen, D.B. (1974) Toward a theory of dream recall. *Psychological Bulletin*, 81, 138-154.

Coles, R. Geological Survey of Canada. Personal communication.

Conesa, J. (1995) Relationship between isolated sleep paralysis and geomagnetic influences: a case study. *Perceptual and Motor Skills*, 80, 1263-1273.

Conesa, J. (1997) Isolated sleep paralysis, vivid dreams and geomagnetic influences: II. *Perceptual and Motor Skills*, 85, 579-584.

Conesa, J. (2000) Geomagnetic, cross-cultural and occupational faces of sleep paralysis: an ecological perspective. *Sleep and Hypnosis*, 2, 105-111.

Conesa, J. (2002) Isolated sleep paralysis and lucid dreaming: ten-year longitudinal case study and related dream frequencies, types, and categories. *Sleep and Hypnosis*, 4 (4), 132-142.

Conesa, J. (2003) Sleep Paralysis Signaling (*SPS*) As A Natural Cueing Method for the Generation and Maintenance of Lucid Dreaming. Presented at The 83rd Annual Convention of the Western Psychological Association, May 1 - 4, 2003 in Vancouver, BC, Canada.

Dawkins, R. (1989) The Selfish Genes (2nd Ed.). Oxford: Oxford University Press.

Delouis, H. and Mayaud, P.N. (1975) Spectral Analysis of the Geomagnetic Activity Index *aa* over a 103-year interval. *Journal of Geophysical Research*, 80, 34, 4681-4688.

Dement, W.C. (1960) The effect of dream deprivation. *Science*, 131,1705-1707.

Dement, W.C., Greenberg, S., Klein, R. (1966) The effect of partial REM sleep deprivation and delayed recovery. *Journal of Experimental Psychology*, 53,339-346.

Dement, W. (1999) The promise of sleep. New York: Delacorte Press.

Diagnostic and Statistical Manual of Mental Disorders, DSM-IV-TR (2000). American Psychiatric Association.

Domhoff, B. (1969) Home dreams versus laboratory dreams. In dream psychology and the new biology of dreaming, ed. M. Kramer. Springfield, Ill: Charles Thomas.

Draper, E.D. (1995) In the doorway. Parabola, Summer 1995, pp.73.

Edinger, E.F. (1995) Melville's Moby Dick: An American Nekyia. Toronto: Inner City Books.

Edinger, E.F. (1973) Ego and archetype: individuation and the religious function of the psyche. Baltimore, Maryland: Penguin Books Inc.

Eliade, M. (1958) Rites and Symbols of Initiation. New York: Harper Torch Books.

Eliade, M. (1964-1951, Fr. Ed.) Shamanism: archaic techniques of ecstasy. New York: Pantheon. (Bollingen Series, LXXVI.)

Eliade, M. (1982) A history of religious ideas, Volume 2. Chicago: University of Chicago Press.

Everett, H.C. (1963) Sleep Paralysis in medical students. *J Nerv Ment Dis.*, 3,283-287.

Firestone, M. (1985) The "Old Hag": sleep paralysis in Newfoundland. *The Journal of Psychoanalytic Anthropology*, 8, 47-66.

Folkard, S., Condon, R., Herbert, M. (1984) Night shift paralysis. *Experimentia*, 40, 510-512.

Folkard, S. and Condon, R. (1987) Night shift paralysis in air traffic control officers. *Ergonomics*, 30, 1353-1363.

Freud, S. (1949-1989) An outline of psychoanalysis. (Translated by James Strachey). New York: Norton & Company.

Freud, S. (1900-1996) The interpretation of dreams. (Translated by A. A. Brill). New York: Random House Value Publishing Inc. (Gracemercy Books).

Friedman, H., Becker, O. and Bachman, C.H. (1965) Psychiatric ward behavior and geophysical parameters. *Nature*, 205, 1050-1052.

Fukuda, K., and Miyasita, A. (1991) Personality of healthy young adults with sleep paralysis. *Perceptual and Motor Skills*,73, 955-962.

Fukuda, K., Miyasita, A., Inugami, M, Ishihara, K. (1987) High prevalence of isolated sleep paralysis: *kanashibari* phenomenon in Japan. *Sleep*,10, 279-286.

Gillis, L. (2002) The Lucid Dream Exchange. Personal Communication (www.dreaminglucid.com.)

Goode, G.B. (1962) Sleep Paralysis. *Archives of Neurology*, 6, 228-234.

Gray, A.A. (1987) Nightmares, hypnagogic hallucinations, and sleep paralysis. In: Kellerman H, (Ed.) The nightmare: psychological and biological foundations, New York: Columbia University Press.

Hall, C., and Van de Castle, R. (1966) The content analysis of dreams. New York: Appleton-Century-Croft.

Hall, C., Van de Castle, R. (1966) Studies of dreams reported in the laboratory and at home. Institute of Dream Research monograph series no.1. California: Big Trees Press.

Hall, C. (1967) Representation of the laboratory setting in dreams. *Journal of Nervous and Mental Disease*, 144,198-206.

Hampden-Turner, (1981) Maps of the mind: Charts and concepts of the mind and its labyrinths. New York: Collier Books/Macmillan Publishing Co., Inc.

Harner, M.J. (1981) Hallucinogens and Shamanism. New York: Oxford University Press.(pp.134.)

Harner, M.J. (1982) The way of the shaman: A guide to power and healing. New York: Bantam Books.

Hartmann, E. (1984) The nightmare: the psychology and biology of terrifying dreams. New York: Basic Books.

Haub, C. (1995) Global and U.S. National Population Trends. *Consequences*, 1, 2.

Hobson, J.A. and McCarley, R. (1977) The brain as a dream-stage generator: activation synthesis hypothesis of the dream process. *American Journal of Psychology*, 134, 1335-1346.

Hobson, J.A. and Stickgold, R. (1994) A neurocognitive approach to dreaming. *Consciousness and Cognition*, 3, 16-29.

Hobson, J.A. and Leonard, J. (2001) Out of its mind: Psychiatry in crisis, a call for reform. New York: Perseus Publishing.

Hoffmeyer, J. (1996) Signs of meaning in the universe. (translated by Barbara J. Haveland). Bloomington: Indiana University Press.

Hofstadter, D.R. and Dennett, D.C. (Eds.) (1981) The mind's I. New York: Basic Books, Inc., Publishers.

Hufford, D.J. (1982) The terror that comes in the night: an experience-centered study of the supernatural assaults traditions. Philadelphia: University of Pennsylvania Press.

Horney, K. (1994) Self analysis. New York: Norton & Company.

Jones, E. (1961) The life and work of Sigmund Freud. New York: Basic Books, Inc.

Johnson, C.P.L. and Persinger, M.A. (1994) The sensed presence may be facilitated by interhemispheric intercalation: relative efficacy of the mind's eye, hemi-synch tape, and bilateral temporal magnetic field stimulation. *Perceptual and Motor Skills*; 79, 351-354.

Jung, C.G. (1956-1976) Symbols of transformation: An analysis of the prelude to a case of schizophrenia. (Translated by R.F.C. Hull) Princeton, N.J.: Princeton University press

Jung, C.G. (Ed.) (1964) Man and his symbols. New York: Dell Publishing Co. Inc.

Jung, C.G. (1976) On America. In George M. Kren and Leon H. Rappoport (Eds.), *Varieties of psychohistory*. New York : Springer Pub. Co.

Keyfitz, N. (1985) Applied mathematical demography (2nd Ed.). New York: Springer-Verlag.

Kleitman, N. (1939) Sleep and wakefulness. Chicago: University of Chicago press.

Kleitman, N. (1960) Patterns of dreaming. *Scientific American*, 203, 81-88.

Kopytenko, Y.A., Komarovskikh, N.I., Voronov, P.M. (1995) Possible link between ultralow frequency electromagnetic lithospheric emissions and the unusual behavior of biological systems before severe earthquakes. *Biophysics*, 40, 1123-1125.

LaBerge S. (1980) Lucid dreaming as a learnable skill: A case study. *Perceptual and Motor Skills*, 51, 1039-1042.

LaBerge S., & Levita L. (1986) Lucid Dreaming: The power of being awake and aware in your dreams. New York: Ballantine Books.

LaBerge S., & Levita L. (1995) Validity established of DreamLight cues for eliciting lucid dreaming. *Dreaming*, 5, 198-206.

LaBerge, S. (2000) Lucid dreaming: Evidence that REM sleep can support unimpaired cognitive function and a methodology for studying the psychophysiology of dreaming. HTML version of LaBerge's (2000) Lucid Dreaming: Evidence and methodology. behavioral and Brain Sciences, (23 (6), 962-963.

LaBerge, S. & DeGracia, D.J. (2000). Varieties of lucid dreaming experience. In R.G. Kunzendorf & B. Wallace (Eds.), Individual Differences in Conscious Experience. Amsterdam: John Benjamins.

Langer, S. (1953) Feeling and form. New York: Charles Scribner's Sons.

Lehn, W.H., and Schroeder, I. (1981) The Norse Merman as an optical phenomenon. *Nature*, 289, 362-366.

Lerchl, A., Honaka, K.O., Reiter, R.J. (1991) Pineal gland 'magnetosensitivity' to static magnetic fields is a consequence of induced electric currents (eddy currents). *Journal of Pineal Research*; 10, 109-116.

Lerchl, A., Reiter, R.J., Howes, K.A., Nokada, K.O., Stokkan, K-A. (1991) Evidence that extremely low frequency Ca2+ -cyclotron resonance depresses pineal melatonin synthesis in vitro. *Neuroscience Letters*, 124, 213-215.

Lévi-Strauss, C. (1962-1966) The savage mind—La Pensee Sauvage. Chicago: The University of Chicago Press.

Lévi-Strauss, C. (1977) Tristes tropiques. (Unabridged translation be John and Doreen Weightman.) New York: Pocket Books.

Llinás, R. (1988) The intrinsic electrophysiological properties of mammalian neurons: Insights into central nervous system function. *Science*, 242, 1654-1664.

Llinás, R. and Pare, D. (1991) Of dreaming and wakefulness. *Neuroscience*, 44, 521-535.

Llinás, R. and Ribary, U. (1993) Coherent 40-Hz oscillation characterizes dream state in humans. *Proc. Natl. Acad. Sci.*, USA, 90, 2078-2081.

Mann, K. and Röschke, J. (1996) Effects of pulsed high-frequency electromagnetic fields on human sleep. *Neuropsychobiology*, 33, 41-7.

Mann, K., Wagner, P., Brunn, G., Hassan, F., Hiemke, C., and Röschke, J. (1998) Effects of pulsed high-frequency electromagnetic fields on the neuroendocrine system. *Neuroendocrinology*, 67, 139-144.

McKay, B.E. and Persinger, M.A. (1999) Geophysical variables and behavior: LXXXVII. Effects of synthetic and natural geomagnetic patterns on maze learning. *Perceptual and Motor Skills*, 89, 1023-1024.

McKellar, P. (1992) Introspective acuity and retrieval: filtering back losses from the dreamlife. *Journal of Mental Imagery*, 16, 167-174.

McKinlay, A. (1997) Possible health effects related to the use of radiotelephones. *Radiological Protection Bulletin*, 187, 9-16.

Metzner, R. (1999) Green Psychology: Transforming our relationship to the earth. Rochester, Vermont: Park Street Press.

Michaud, L.Y. and Persinger, M.A. (1985) Geophysical variables and behavior: XXV. Alterations in memory for a narrative following application of theta frequency electromagnetic fields. *Perceptual and Motor Skills*, 60, 416-418.

Mitchell, S.W. (1876) On some of the disorders of sleep. *Virginia Med. Mth.*, 2, 769-781.

Monroe, R.A. (1977) Journeys out of the body. New York: AnchorPress/Doubleday.

Murillo, M. Sleep paralysis and heart attacks. Personal communication.

Naranjo, C. (1967) Psychotropic properties of the harmala alkaloids. In Daniel H. Efron (Ed.) Ethnopharmacologic Search for Psychoactive Drugs. *Public Health Service Publication 1645*. Washington, D.C.: U.S. department of Health, Education and Welfare.

Nardi, T.J. (1981) Treating sleep paralysis with hypnosis. *The International J. Clincl. and Expimntl. Hypno.*, XXV, 4, 358-365.

Ness, R.C. (1978) "The Old Hag" phenomenon as sleep paralysis: a bicultural interpretation. *Culture, Medicine and Psychiatry*, 2,15-39.

Newman, J. and Baars, B.J. (1993) A neural attentional model for access to consciousness: a global workspace perspective. *Concepts in Neuroscience*, 4, 2, 255-290.

Newman, J. (1995) Review: Thalamic contributions to attention and consciousness. *Consciousness & Cognition*, 4, 2.

Nietzche, F.W. (1909) Human, all too human. (translated by Helen Zimmern and Paul Cohn) and published in London was Jung's reference found in a different format in Nietzche, F.W (1986) Human, All Too Human: A Book for Free Spirits. In (Translated by. R. J. Hollingdale from *Menschlich, Allzumenschliches*: Erste Band, 1878.). Cambridge: Cambridge University Press.

O'Connor, R.P. and Persinger, M.A. (1997) Geophysical variables and behavior: LXXXII. A strong association between sudden infant death syndrome and increments of global geomagnetic activity—possible support for the melatonin hypothesis. *Perceptual and Motor Skills*, 84, 395-402.

Ohaeri, J.U., Odejide, A.O., Ikuesan, B.A., Adeyemi, J.D. (1989) The pattern of isolated sleep paralysis among Nigerian medical students. *Journal of the National Medical Association*, 81, 805-808.

Ohaeri, J.U., Adelekan, M.F., Odejide, A.O., Ikuesa, B.A. (1992) The pattern of isolated sleep paralysis among Nigerian nursing students. *Journal of the National medical Association*, 84:67:70

Ohayon, M.M., Zulley, J., Guilleminault, C., Smirne, S. (1999) Prevalence and pathologic associations of sleep paralysis in the general population. *Neurology*, 52:1194:1200.

Ornstein, R.E. (1977) The psychology of consciousness, 2nd Ed. New York: Harcourt Brace Jovanovich, Inc.

Ortega y Gasset, J. (1958-1962) Man and crisis. New York: W.W. Norton & Company, Inc.(pp.14.)

Payn, S.B. (1965) A psychoanalytic approach to sleep paralysis: review and report of a case. *J. Nerv. Ment. Dis.*, 140, 427-433.

Penn, N.E., Kripke, D.F., Scharff, J. (1981) Sleep paralysis among medical students. *Journal of Psychology*, 107, 247-252.

Persinger, M.A. (1985) Geophysical variables and behavior: XXII. The tectonogenic strain continuum of unusual events. *Perceptual and Motor Skills*, 60, 59-65.

Persinger, M.A. (1985) Geophysical variables and behavior: XXX. Intense paranormal experiences occur during days of quiet, global, geomagnetic activity. *Perceptual and Motor Skills*, 61, 320-322.

Persinger, M.A. and Cameron, R.A. (1986) Are earth faults at fault in some poltergeist-like episodes? *The Journal of The American Society for Psychical Research*, 80, 49-73.

Persinger, M.A. (1987) Geopsychology and geopsychopathology: mental processes and disorders associated with geochemical and geophysical factors. *Experientia*, 43, 92-103.

Persinger, M.A. (1988) Increased geomagnetic activity and the occurrence of bereavement hallucinations: evidence for melatonin-mediated microseizuring in the temporal lobe? *Neuroscience Letters*, 88, 271-274.

Persinger, M.A. (1989) Geophysical variables and behavior: LV. predicting the details of visitor experiences and the personality of experiments: the temporal lobe factor. *Perceptual and Motor Skills*, 68, 55-65.

Randall, W. and Randall S. (1991) The solar wind hallucinations- A possible relation due to magnetic disturbances. *Bioelectromagnetics*, 12, 67-70.

Reiter, R.J. and Richardson, B.A. (1992) Magnetic field effects on pineal indoleamine metabolism and possible biological consequences. *The FASEB Journal*, 6, 2283-2287.

Reiter, R.J. (1993) A review of neuroendocrine and neurochemical changes associated with static and extremely low frequency electromagnetic field exposure. *Integrative Physiological and Behavioral Science*, 28, 57-75.

Roszak, T. (1992) *The voice of the earth*. New York: Simon & Schuster.

Sandyk, R. (1997) Resolution of sleep paralysis by weak electromagnetic fields in a patient with multiple sclerosis. *Int. J. Neurosci.*, 90, 145-157.

Schneck, J.M. (1948) Sleep paralysis, psychodynamics. *Psychiatric Quarterly*, 22, 462-464.

Schneck, J.M. (1952) Sleep paralysis. *Am. J. Psychiatry*, 108, 921-923.

Schneck, J.M. (1957) Sleep paralysis, a new evaluation. *Dis. Nerv. Syst.*, 18, 144-146.

Schneck, J.M. (1960) Sleep paralysis without narcolepsy or cataplexy. *J. Amer. Med. Ass.*, 173, 1129-1130.

Schneck, J.M. (1961) Sleep paralysis. *Psychosomatics*, 2, 360-361.

Schneck, J.M. (1966) Narcolepsy, cataplexy, sleep paralysis and hypnagogic hallucinations. In H.F. Conn, R.J. Clohecy and R.B. Conn, Jr. (Eds.), Current Diagnosis. Philadelphia: Saunders.

Schneck, J.M. (1969) Personality components in patients with sleep paralysis. *Psychiatr. Quart.*, 43, 343-348.

Schneck, J.M. (1977) Sleep paralysis and microsomatognosia with special reference to hypnotherapy. *The International Journal of Clinical and Experimental Hypnosis*, XXV, 72-77.

Schredl, M. and Ealacher, D. (2003) The problem of dream content analysis validity as shown by a bizarreness scale. *Sleep and Hypnosis*, 5, 3, 129-135.

Searle, J.R. (1994) The problem of consciousness. In A. Revonsuo and M. Kamppinen (Eds.). Consciousness in philosophy and cognitive neuroscience (pp. 93-104). N.J.: Erlbaum.

Semm, P., Schneider, T., Vollrath, L. (1980) Effects of an Earth-strength magnetic field on electrical activity of pineal cells. *Nature*, 288, 607-608.

Shannon, B. (2003) Altered states and the study of consciousness: The case of ayahuaska. The Journal of Mind and Behavior, 24, 2, 125-154.

Shepard, P. (1998) Nature and Madness. London: The University of Georgia Press.

Snyder, S. (1983) Isolated sleep paralysis after rapid time zone change—'jet lag'—syndrome. *Chronobiologia*, 10, 377-379.

Spanos, N.P., Cross, P.A., Dickson, K., DuBreuil, S.C. (1993) Close encounters: an examination of UFO experiences. *Journal of Abnormal Psychology*, 102, 624-632.

Spanos, N. P.,. McNulty, S.A., DuBreuil, S.C., Pires, M., Burgess, M.F. (1995) The frequency and correlates of sleep paralysis in a university sample. *Journal of Research in Personality*, 29, 3, 285-305.

Stewart, K. (1969) Dream theory in Malaya. In Charles T. Tart (Ed.) Altered States of Consciousness. New York: Doubleday Anchor Book. 161-170.

Takeshi, I. and Akifumi T. (1999) How could neural networks represent higher cognitive functions?: A computational model based on a fractal neural network The Second International Conference on Cognitive Science and The 16th Annual Meeting of the Japanese Cognitive Science Society Joint Conference (ICCS/JCSS99).

Takeshi, I. and Akifumi T. (1999) Modularity and Hierarchy: The Fractal Theory of Consciousness based on the Fractal Neural Network. *Toward a Science of Consciousness*, TOKYO '99.

Takeshi, I. and Akifumi T. (1999) Modularity and Hierarchy in the Cerebral Cortex: A Proposal of Fractal Neural Network. Neural Networks in Applications NN '99, Proceedings of the Fourth International Workshop, 23-29.

Takeuchi T, Miyasita Y, Sasaki Y, Inugami M, Fukuda K. (1992) Isolated sleep paralysis elicited by sleep interruption. *American Sleep Disorders Association and Sleep Research Society*, 15, 217-225.

Takeuchi T, Miyasita Y, Inugami M, Sasaki Y, Fukuda K. (1993) Laboratory-documented hallucination during sleep-onset REM period in a normal subject. *Perceptual and Motor Skills*, 78:217:225.

Takeuchi, T., Miyasita, A., Inugami, M. & Yamamoto, Y. (2001). Intrinsic dreams are not produced without REM sleep mechanisms: evidence through elicitation of sleep onset REM periods. *Journal of Sleep Research*, 10, 1, 43.

Takeuchi, T., Fukuda, K., Sasaki, Y., Inugami, M., Murphy, T. (2002) Factors related to the occurrence of isolated sleep paralysis elicited during a multi-phasic sleep-wake schedule. *Sleep*, 25, 1, 89-96.

Takeuchi, T., Ogilve, R.D., Murphy, T., & Ferrelli A.V. (2003) EEG activities during elicited sleep onset REM and NREM periods reflect different mechanisms of dream generation. *Clinical Neurophysiology*, 114, 210-220.

Tart, C.T. (Ed.) Altered States of Consciousness. New York: Doubleday Anchor Book.

Van Der Hede, C. and Weinbreg, J. (1945) Sleep paralysis and combat fatigue. *Psychosomatic Medicine*, 7, 330-334.

Van Eeden, F. (1913) A study of dreams. *Pro. Soc. Psych. Res.*, 26, 431-461.

Van Eeden, F. (1918) The bridge of dreams. New York: Mitchell Kennerly.

Van de Castle, R.L. (1994) Our dreaming mind. New York: Ballantine Books.

Villoresi, G., Breus, T.K., Dorman, L.I., Iucci, N. (1995) Effect of interplanetary and geomagnetic disturbance on the rise in the number of clinically severe pathologies. *Biophysics*, 40, 983-993.

Wasson, R.G. (1983) Soma divine mushroom of immortality. New York: A Harvest/Harcourt brace Jovanovich, Inc.

Wilson, B.W., Stevens, R.G., Anderson, L.E. (1989) Neuroendocrine mediated effects of electromagnetic field exposure: possible role of the pineal gland. *Life Sciences*, 49, 85-92.

Wilson, S.A.K. (1928) The narcolepsies. *Brain*, 51, 63-109.

Wing, Y.K, Lee, S.T., Chen, C.N. (1994) Sleep paralysis in Chinese: ghost oppression phenomenon in Hong Kong. *Sleep*, 17, 609-613.

Wing, Y.K, Chiu, H., Leung, T., Ng, J. (1999) Sleep paralysis in the elderly. *J. Sleep Res.*, 8, 151-155.

Wolpin, M., Marston, A., Randolph, C., Clothier, A. (1992)

Individual difference correlates of reported lucid dreaming frequency and control. *Journal of Mental Imagery*, 16, 231-236.

Yaga, K., Reiter, R.J., Manchester, L., Nieves, H., Sun, J-H., Chen, L-D. (1993) Pineal sensitivity to pulsed static magnetic fields changes during photoperiod. *Brain Research Bulletin*, 30, 153-156.

Zinberg, N.E. (Ed.) (1977) Alternate state of consciousness: Multiple perspectives on the study of consciousness. New York: The Free Press/Macmillan Publishing Co., Inc.

Printed in the United States
222205BV00001B/14/A